CROHN'S INTERRUPTED:
Living Life Triumphantly

To

Brutha War.

I hope my story inspired you.

Peace & Blessings

MAW

11/3/17

This book is not intended or implied to be a substitute for professional medical advice, diagnosis or treatment. The reader should regularly consult a physician in matters relating to his/her health and particularly with respect to any symptoms that may require diagnosis or medical attention. All content in this book is for general information purposes only. In the event you use this information without your doctor's approval, you are prescribing for yourself, which is your constitutional right, but the publisher and the author assume no responsibility.

About the Author

Makeda Armorer-Wade is a dynamic and influential leader who has become an expert in managing life as a Crohn's Survivor. She has 30 + years of experience gracefully managing and battling the tragic diagnosis of Crohn's disease since she was 16 years old. Life has provided unlimited opportunities for her, to tame this beast called Crohn's. Ms. Armorer-Wade has developed a full wheat, corn, yeast and dairy free diet, along with discovering new ways to make breads and desserts that have become alternative food sources. Ms. Armorer-Wade holds a MS in Human Services Administration and an MSW with a Specialization in Children and Family Counseling. She has been in the field of Social Services for over twenty-five (25) years and believes in giving back. She serves as Trustee, 2nd Vice President and Membership Chair of the Schomburg Corporation, as well as participates on the Executive Board for her chapter in Alpha Kappa Alpha Sorority, Inc.

Currently she is a Curriculum Developer for the City of New York where she has written over 15 curricula. She also serves as the Chief Strategist at Chiron Enterprises. Ms. Armorer-Wade has a passion for teaching that has led her to be an online Instructor for Axia College now University of Phoenix, an Instructor at Fordham University and a Trainer for the City of New York. And if that wasn't enough in 2002, she started a non-profit called Mentors on the Move, Inc. where she began mentoring and coaching young women on a variety of issues. In all areas especially with the young women she mentors she promotes "Taking the best and leaving the rest." Ms. Armorer-Wade also serves as a member and on the Executive Board of GAYAP Incorporated and participated in fundraising to support orphanages internationally.

Ms. Armorer-Wade attributes her strong faith to triumphantly winning this life long battle against Crohn's Disease. She is a proud wife and parent of three talented young men, Jason, Jaron and Jafari.

Contents

*There is nothing
Small about you*

*You have a mighty soul,
an important purpose and a
unique gift to give to this world.*

*Playing small doesn't serve you,
your creator, or the world who
needs your light.*

*Give yourself Permission to play
a bigger game*

*And watch as the universe con-
spires to assist you.*
- Mastinkipp.com

PREFACE

"Things turn out best for those that make the best of how things turn out." There have not been any patients that I have cared for over the past 25 years that have followed this verdict more than Makeda Armorer-Wade. When I first met Makeda, she had already been through a great deal. First diagnosed with Crohn's in her teenage years, she had numerous surgeries early on in her course of disease due to repeated intestinal obstructions and other complications of her aggressive disease. During my initial consultation with Makeda in the office, I knew that her illness was very complex, and her struggles to prevent recurrent complications of Crohn's would be challenging.

However, despite seeing how her illness has progressed, I am constantly struck by her sincere smile in the face of often feeling lousy and her ability to look forward. Instead of harping on the harrowing symptoms that she feels on a daily basis, she looks to the future with optimism, always asking what steps we can take to make her situation better. Crohn's disease is an inflammatory condition of the gastrointestinal tract. It can affect any part of the intestine from the mouth to the anus. Unfortunately the cause has not yet been elucidated, and there is no cure. There is a very wide spectrum of disease presentation. Some patients with Crohn's have mild abdominal pain and diarrhea, and can be managed with dietary changes and small doses of oral medications. However, others have severe disease that may lead to obstruction and intestinal bleeding; these cases frequently require more aggressive anti-inflammatory medications, frequently by intravenous infusion or injection.

Often times this inflammation can be nonresponsive to medication and require surgery. Makeda's disease has been very aggressive.

She has required countless medication changes along the way and has undergone many surgeries. Since her first surgery very early on as a young girl, fortunately, there have been many advances made in the treatment of Crohn's disease. In the past 5 years, she has received several of the latest medications that target the immune response in an attempt to control intestinal inflammation. However, numerous times, her disease did not respond to these drugs. Through all of this hardship and despite some of her surgeries resulting in complications such as wound infections, her positive attitude and her smile shines through with every office visit. In addition, her fierce determination to move forward with life's activities has been evident. Frequently, she would schedule her office visit early in the morning so she could keep her full day at work. There are times when I wonder how anyone could handle the difficulties she has been going through on a daily basis, from abdominal pain to uncontrollable diarrhea, or when she faced drainage from her surgical wounds.

She not only gets through her day, she does it without complaining, not even to the office staff. I often marvel at her courage, seeing how sick she is at times, yet never letting that interfere with her daily routines. During one of her severe Crohn's flares, she consulted with a colleague of mine who is also a specialist in the field of Crohn's disease, to see if she may benefit from any experimental medications prior to considering surgery. When he called me after the visit, his first comment was how extraordinary this person is to be fighting this illness so gracefully. I often remarked to my office staff that many other patients with her complications would be on disability rather than maintaining full time employment. It makes me think all the patients I have who ask for notes to be excused from work who have not been nearly as ill as Makeda, yet she has never requested an absence note. In addition to the positive outlook and amazing perseverance, Makeda has always been prepared for the next step. Due to the complex nature of her Crohn's phenotype, she has had a lot of next steps!!! I often wonder prior to walking in the office how she is going to deal with the news that this promising new medication is not working. But there was never a "Why me?" or "I can't believe this is happening again." Instead what I heard was "OK, so what's next? How can we make this better?" With Makeda there is no looking back at the past; it's about going forward. At each step of the way, it is also working as a team to figure out a new approach when the last one failed. Makeda never sat around and waited. Once we formulate a plan together, she is her own advocate, frequently making the calls, whether to the insurance company to fight for drug approval or arranging dates and times for infusion medication. In addition to the conventional medications for her illness, Makeda has always been proactive in maintaining proper nutrition. I have witnessed her focus on maintaining a very strict diet. Although our medical literature is lacking in studies to determine the best diet for Crohn's disease, Makeda has made it part of her mission to research nutritional therapies and find specific nutritionists with a background in Crohn's disease. In fact, I have incorporated some of what she has done with her diet to help my other Crohn's patients feel better and live healthier lives. Makeda is one of the few patients I have cared for that has left a strong impact on my career. She has an amazing ability to persevere through a very difficult chronic illness, and has done so with Grace and dignity. I do believe that her approach to fighting her complex disease will not only help her cope, but also will help so many other people who struggle with similar chronic illnesses. As her gastroenterologist, I feel blessed to be able to have taken care of her over the years, and look forward to assisting in keeping her well in the future.

Dr. Robert Rosenzweig

Introduction

Let me tell you a story about a vital intelligent, engaged and responsible young lady. She had a lively personality, was athletic - involved in every sport you can think of both personally and as a spectator – inclined to play with the boys as much as with the girls. She was intellectually curious and devoted to scholarship.

She had no idea, absolutely no idea that when she didn't feel well that November day that it would begin an odyssey of 30 plus years 17 surgeries and hundreds of doctor visits that would bring her to where she is today.

It all started one Thanksgiving, she was looking forward to the usual family feast, but she started to feel ill. She had an uncharacteristic sharp abdominal pain and no appetite. She began running a temperature of 102. The family consulted with the doctor and she was told to take Tylenol and come in on Monday. That Monday the doctor said it was an infection and treated her with antibiotics. They admitted her into the hospital and were prepared to do surgery when the pain disappeared. The doctor's stated that the appendix must have ruptured and they could treat with antibiotics and operate at a later date. This went on for several months, a cycle of pain, fever, Tylenol, antibiotics over and over. One day while her father was at the dentist he mentioned his concerns and the dentist immediately offered to send them over to his brother who was a general practitioner. He examined her and he called a friend of his who was a surgeon. Within hours after that appointment she was admitted to the hospital having identified that she had an abscess on the wall of her side, diagnosis: peritonitis. They decided to do surgery right away. Once they completed that surgery the infection seemed to explode it became uncontrollable. They could not keep it contained. Her parents were told to go home and get their papers in order because she wasn't going to make it. Instead of planning a sweet 16 party she was given a death sentence.

This poor girl was in isolation because they said any possible organism could impact her health. The diagnosis stumped her doctors. Her symptoms defied all characterization Healing would take place in one section of her gastro intestinal tract only to have the symptoms recur in a different area the symptomology was not relative to her demographic. The doctors could make no sense of it. The closest diagnosis was more relative to descendants of Mediterranean or Jewish cultures. This did not relate to her.

Family and friends were terrified for her life, she couldn't eat and had declined to a mere 78 pounds and was extremely frail. Sixteen was too young to die! However her only concern was keeping up with her homework and studies because she wanted to live; live to take the New York State Regents exams so she could attend college. She continued to believe that she would be okay even when the nurses said don't bother doing homework you need to enjoy your last days! Defying all odds, they decided to send her home from the hospital feeling that she would have a better quality of life for her remaining days. She had a six inch open wound on her stomach that had to be irrigated and packed twice a day. Most patients would have a visiting nurse to handle this delicate procedure, not this young lady; she had them teach her how to do it and mastered doing it herself. Once she demonstrated her ability to do this on her own they let her do it. What was not apparent to others at the time was her motive for this; because of her sense of independence and determination she gave herself the ability to return to school quicker. The school could not believe that she was walking around with a wound that large on her side. Who does that? When she returned to school, they were astonished by the show of strength because she used to walk with a cane due to the severe weight loss. The ligaments in her knees had shrunk and could not support her weight.

This young lady was determined to sit for the Regents exams her last year of high school. She passed them all and went on to receive her general diploma and Regents Diploma. Again her doctors recommended that she rest and delay starting college. She refused because her position was that she can stay home and be in pain or she can go to school in pain, but time is going to pass anyway so she might as well have accomplished something. She did compromise though and went to Herbert H. Lehman College of the City University locally so that she could be close to her doctors. She was determined to be as normal as possible. Can you believe this was me?

Talking about Crohn's Disease is not anything I ever wanted to do publicly or otherwise. As a young person I always felt ashamed of having it although I had no control over the constant bathroom runs and daily exhaustion. Several people including my Gastroenterologist have encouraged me to document my story in hopes that It might provide encouragement and hope to someone else (notice that I did not say in the same situation, because no two are alike). I have always been a firm believer in keeping your business private, and that's why it's called personal business; but as I move through this life, I have come to the realization that so many people have so many different life issues. You never know why people comport themselves in the manner that they do. Different people observing me would not really understand what was going on many times. So rather than ask, why me? I asked God to use me in a way that will benefit others who suffer from some of the same afflictions that I had and still do. I will be a Servant Leader. You will find that I will give you the 'real deal' about things, but then I will reframe to always look at the positive lesson or message that I received. A little Pollyanna you may think, but it makes a huge difference in the quality of your life. I have the expectation that I am going to land on my feet so when I stumble, because I expect to land on my feet, I put my feet down. It's a conscious decision.

My main goal in life is to not only manage my own symptoms and enjoy participating in my life but to inspire Crohn's patients and my fellow Ostomates (Ostomates-, those having a urostomy, colostomy or ileostomy) to understand and believe that life is not over based on their situation. They can live a full and enjoyable life despite their diagnosis. They have to acknowledge that there will be obstacles to go over, under and around but it can be done, once you make up your mind to fight for your life.

At this time Crohn's may be a life sentence, but it does not have to be a death sentence. You have to be able to dream the possibility in order to plan to achieve it. You can do it and I can help you.

What is Crohn's Disease?

Crohn's Disease can be a life threatening debilitating life thief. It is an embarrassing difficult disease that can tear your life and your family's life apart. There are many types of Crohn's Disease and various ways that it can affect your body. The disease can form anywhere from your throat all the way through to your colon. I have experienced it in my small intestine, large intestine and lower bowel.

Let me give you the medical definition so that you can better understand how this disease functions.

"Crohn's disease is a chronic inflammatory bowel disease (IBD) characterized by inflammation. Immune response to tissue injury that causes redness, swelling, and pain of the digestive, or gastrointestinal (GI) tract, collectively referring to;

the mouth, esophagus, stomach, small and large intestines, and anus. In fact, Crohn's can affect any part of the GI tract, from the mouth to the anus but it is more commonly found at the end of the small intestine (A long, tube-like organ in the abdomen that completes the process of digestion). It consists of the small and large intestines. Also called the bowel (the ileum) where it joins the beginning of the large intestine (or colon). It can also affect: eyes, skin and joints. (Understanding Crohn's Disease, 2016)

Crohn's Disease vs. Ulcerative Colitis

Both Crohn's Disease and Ulcerative Colitis (UC) are inflammatory bowel diseases (IBDs), but there are some key differences.

Crohn's Disease
Inflammation may develop anywhere in the GI tract from the mouth to the anus

- Most commonly occurs at the end of the small intestine
- May appear in patches
- May extend through entire thickness of bowel wall
- About 67% of people in remission will have at least 1 relapse over the next 5 years

Ulcerative Colitis
- Limited to the large intestine (colon and rectum)
- Occurs in the rectum and colon, involving a part or the entire colon

- Appears in a continuous pattern
- Inflammation occurs in innermost lining of the intestine
- About 30% of people in remission will experience a relapse in the next year
- IBD is not IBS

It's important not to confuse an inflammatory bowel disease (IBD) like Crohn's disease or ulcerative colitis with irritable bowel syndrome (IBS). IBS is a disorder that affects the muscle contractions of the bowel and is not characterized by intestinal inflammation, nor is it a chronic disease.

Currently there are 700,000 people who are diagnosed with Crohn's Disease. Men and women alike. It can occur at any time but is usually diagnosed between 15 and 35. Symptoms range from mild to severe.

Crohn's disease symptoms range from

mild to severe. They may vary over time and from person to person, depending on what part of the gastrointestinal (GI) tract. Collectively referring to the mouth, esophagus, stomach, small and large intestines, and anus. Is inflamed. And because symptoms vary from person to person, the way to gauge what you consider a flare-up of symptoms is relative to what is "normal" for you. (Understanding Crohn's Disease, 2016)

Common Crohn's disease symptoms include:
- Frequent, recurring diarrhea
- Rectal Lowest portion of the large intestine that connects to the anus. bleeding
- Unexplained weight loss
- Fever
- Abdominal pain and cramping
- Fatigue and a feeling of low energy
- Reduced appetite

Crohn's can affect the entire GI tract — from the mouth to the anus — and can be progressive increasing in extent or severity, so over time your symptoms could get worse. That's why it's important that you have an open and honest conversation about your symptoms, since your doctor will use that information to help determine what treatment plan is best for you.

It might be helpful to refer to the chart below to help you understand the differences between mild, moderate and severe symptoms, since your doctor may use similar measures.

Crohn's Disease Symptom Severity

You may have symptoms such as:

- Frequent diarrhea
- Abdominal pain (but can walk and eat normally)
- Possible signs of:
    - o Dehydration
    - o High fever
    - o Abdominal tenderness
    - o Painful mass
    - o Intestinal obstruction
    - o Weight loss of more than 10%

Moderate to Severe

You may have symptoms such as:
- Frequent diarrhea
- Abdominal pain or tenderness
- Fever
- Significant weight loss
- Significant anemia (a few of these symptoms may include fatigue, shortness of breath, dizziness and headache)

Very Severe

Persistent symptoms despite appropriate treatment for moderate to severe Crohn's, and you may also experience:
- High fever
- Persistent vomiting
- Evidence of intestinal obstruction (blockage) or abscess (localized infection or collection of pus). A few of these symptoms may include abdominal pain that doesn't go away or gets worse, swelling of the abdomen, nausea or vomiting, diarrhea, and constipation.
- More severe weight loss

Once you and your doctor have discussed your symptoms and created a treatment plan, it's important to follow directions and take your treatment as prescribed. If you ever have any questions or concerns about your treatment, you should contact your doctor before making any changes or adjustments.
Crohn's disease is unpredictable.

Over time, your symptoms may change in severity, or change altogether. You may go through periods of remission— when you have few or no symptoms, or your symptoms may come on suddenly, without warning.
(Crohn's Symptoms, 2016)

Medications:
 There are many different types of medications that are prescribed for Crohn's Disease. The following are just a few that I know of:
- Asacol,
- Dicyclomine,
- MP6,
- Cimzia,

- Humira,
- Remicade,
- Entyvio
- Cipro,
- Methatraxolone and the list is growing.

Some of these medications can have very severe side effects. If you find that you are experiencing any changes contact your doctor. If you are the care giver or family member and you notice drastic changes in the patient do not dismiss it. Contact their medical provider for instructions.

Inspiration

Having a Crohn's Disease diagnosis can be quite scary and depressing. It can be very different for each person battling the disease. You can make a choice to whine, complain and give up or handle it with dignity and Grace. Actually I support both approaches, but every pity party should be timed. (I will discuss that later). I am writing this book as a labor of love and to be an inspiration to those of you who struggle with Crohn's Disease and resulting Ostomies, and for those of you who are the loved ones affected by the illness: spouses, parents, siblings, caretakers and friends.

I watched my mother go through many hardships and she always handled things with dignity and Grace. So I chose to follow her example. I made her rules mine; I keep my head up and put a welcoming smile on my face.

Many days I've woken up to severe pain, stomach cramps and vomiting from the disease and/or the medication. The hardest part is the uncertainty of knowing what each day or flare up of the disease will bring. The difficulty in being unable to make solid plans in the present or in the future or making plans and not being able to fulfill your commitments to others.

Managing the disappointment of others when you inform them that you cannot attend an event or participate in a planned activity can be tough, but managing your own disappointment can be more difficult. People don't under-stand that you can be fine today and complete-ly debilitated the next. Many of us suffer with diarrhea or constipation, cramps or vomiting. We are never really sure of what each day will hold.

So I programmed myself to take the best and leave the rest. Living one day at a time is enough. I play the gratitude game with myself giving thanks for every little thing that happens daily. It goes something like this. I wake up and say I am grateful. I can get out of the bed on my own; I say I am grateful. I stand up and stretch and go to the bathroom by myself; I am grateful. I can brush my teeth and get dressed without assis-tance; I am grateful. I can prepare my breakfast; I am grateful. I can sit to drive myself to work; I am grateful. I can walk from where I parked to the building and make it to my desk; I am grateful, and this is how my day goes because I remember so many days when none of those tasks were possible. Gratitude allows me to function and avoid being stressed about what I am unable to do; and some days that's a lot.

My approach is to always do my best and work to forgive myself for the times when my best is not good enough or doesn't meet the mark by my standard. I always strive for excellence. According to my sister she always asks how I am feeling, and when I respond 'ok' she asks is that a Makeda ok or really ok? I ask what does that mean and she explained that when I say it's a regular ok, it means I'm facing normal levels of challenges but when it's a Makeda level of ok everyone else would be knocked out from the distress.

It's not only information that I want to share but the inspiration. I want to inspire my fellow Crohn's patients and Ostomates to embrace their "new" normal life.

YOU have to set the standard. The struggle is real, but how you manage it can be the difference between depression, and being a shut in and choosing to live; and by living I mean a life where you feel productive; a life where you can go out and enjoy yourself; a life where you can continue to work and contribute. I literally have to fight this disease daily just to go to work. Many days I am told that I could be on disability if I wanted to because people with much less serious issues were declared totally disabled, but working maintains my sense of self. It gives me dignity and allows me to thumb my nose at Crohn's. It gives me something great to look forward to and an opportunity where I can help others. I love writing curricula and interacting with my colleagues. I work hard to tame this beast called Crohn's continuously, but writing allows me to contribute and share my experience with others indirectly, and hopefully impact the lives of children and adults in a positive manner. This is what I was born to do. When I feel well enough, I max out every opportunity for fun. I love to dance roller skate and enjoy life, so when I get the chance I make it my business to enjoy every note of every song. As Prince's song says "Party like its 1999". I will not compromise on any day where I can physically express my love for life. I remember not being able to make it more than half a block without stopping to breathe. So often we take life, independence and mobility for granted. However, when you can't take care of yourself or be independently mobile you gain a completely different perspective on life.

You don't know what it means to be well until you get sick; especially if you don't know whether or not you will ever get better. If you break your leg, you know at some point you're going to heal. The bones will mend and you will be able to use your leg again. But with a chronic illness it is unpredictable. You never know if you'll ever get better.

My friends, family and Doctor's know me well enough to understand that I am not going to quit. I figure if I am going to be in pain, I can pack up the pain with me and go out and see what life is offering that day. I have come to learn that what other people think about me is none of my business (except compliments – those I take personally). I like me, so if others like me that's a bonus.

Guiding Principles

Lisa Nichols says: "There is a divine calling on your life, and you have to own it." (Nichols, 2016) This statement resonated to my core. She said "You don't have the right to keep your gift to yourself. God gave it to you so you can help someone else." (Nichols, 2016)

God's going to give you what you can handle in this moment now. I've really gone through some tough stuff; I've had my days and weeks where my goal for the day was to not wake up in pain. I've had months where all I wanted to do was find a little bit of joy in between the pressure and pain.

I've had times where I wanted to be proud of the woman I had become and I wasn't because I was hunched over and walking likes a 90 year old in constant need of assistance. Not that there is anything wrong with a 90 year old but I am not 90. I remember not being able to walk; I would come home from work and sit in my car for 20 minutes because I did not have the strength to get out. I remember not being able to lie down, sleep or sit without pain. I would often have the conversation of "why me?" and then I would answer "why not me". Being in severe pain caused me to isolate myself sometimes because I found that although my friends and family loved and supported me they could not handle seeing me in that kind of pain. Sometimes I honestly did not have the strength to engage or even put on my brave front. I couldn't fake "alrightness".

Sometimes I wanted to ask strangers if I could just hold onto them for them to tow me one block to my car because I couldn't breathe. One of the side effects of my many surgeries was having pulmonary emboli (P.E).'s in both lungs and deep vein thrombosis (DVT) in my leg.

I am convinced there is a Divine calling

for my life. I had to learn that I was not going through these unbearable experiences alone but that God was bringing me through them. I was a walking, talking, breathing miracle in the making. God was going to use my life to help somebody else.

When I was told by the doctors that there was nothing more that they could do, I was being set up for the next miracle. This is the next best season in my life. Lisa says "You don't put a period where a comma is supposed to be. You don't get to opt out on the calling that your life was created to share". (Nichols, 2016) Upon hearing this, my first thought was "but I am a private person". It took a lot for me to recognize that I was created with the resiliency, perseverance, tenacity and blind unwavering faith that would be an example for others. The only way I made it through was trusting in God and exercising my faith to see the other side while I was going through it. I had to be able to look down the road and know it would be alright. I had to ask "what am I going to do with this lesson?" The answer was You are going to help people heal. You are going to help them see the possibility for their life. You are going to help them understand that these adversities and resulting lessons are a "gift wrapped in sandpaper". (Nichols, 2016)

So I am rising above it not standing in it. That thing that knocked me down gave me my biggest pause, over and over. When I went down, I landed on my backside so I could look up and give praise for the miracle that I knew was about to happen.

I have learned to frame my challenges as God wanting me to see the greatness that he created in me. I was told that the calling on my life had more to do with someone who is going to cross my path. Someone that really needs me is going to come into my life. YOU can't contain what your about to do. Lisa Nichols said and I believe "Don't let your yesterday limit your tomorrow, your next week...just put a comma on it not a period." I was asked are you willing to stand up to the chance of being seen and/or heard or speak up at the chance of somebody listening; are you going to show up at the chance that somebody is going to show up with you and for you. I used to be the Lone Ranger, - you know that person that believes that they can do it all on their own. And I had to learn that it was alright to ask for help when I needed it; that the Universe would hear me and send all that I needed. I had been let down in the past and didn't trust people to really understand or come through for me. I felt like other than my family I was the only one that I could trust not to let me down. I had to confront my past in order to set up my future to let someone in. When you are going through the challenge you need to pause for a minute. Lisa Nichols says "Don't take out real estate in your pause." God says that this too shall pass. "You have to get back up and understand that you are your own rescue. You with your experiences can help someone to rescue themselves. No one can talk, act or say it like you. Everything that you have gone through has set you up for this". (Nichols, 2016)

I didn't go through it, I was brought through it. I refuse to land and stay on the experience. God has brought me through it each and every time. I've been brought through trying to do it all by myself. It's easy to talk about it now and it's time to step up and step into a new life, do things differently. By asking for what I needed, I began to get endless support. I was told you are only making withdrawals on the deposits that you made into the bank of other's lives. They told me they were waiting for me to figure out that I didn't need to be so independent and do it all on my own.

Lisa Nichols said someone somewhere needs to see you and witness what it looks like to get knocked down and get back up with Grace. What it looks like to love my body with all of my battle wounds and witness what it looks like to press reset and give yourself another chance. My life is about you crossing my path.

I am willing because God said he would never leave me or forsake me. Greater is he than he who is in me than he who is in the world. (1 John 4:4) Where the demand is, you will provide the supply. I believe it to be so. When you really choose to believe, you are saying that you believe in the absence of any physical evidence. I believe in the absence of seeing what I am believing. This is why I have been able to press forward regardless of what my medical team sees as my limits. They are often amazed at how I cope and ask for tips that they can share with their patients. They ask to use my stories like the bathroom in my car or managing others disclosures to me. That's called unwavering faith. You simply cannot have faith requiring evidence. You just cannot have faith requiring evidence. Faith asks can you be joyful, give praise and see the possibility in midst of the storm. I say yes I am the living breathing, walking, talking miracle that you see before you. The proof that you need.

God says can you stand up for yourself today. I woke up to my possibility. Can I give myself a chance to be great? Absolutely! Can I not dumb down or play small to make others feel powerful? Today, I give myself the chance to be exactly who God designed me to be. I am no longer asking permission, I am giving notice.

I am not someone who is in a heap of mess but someone who has a divine message because of my struggles with my illness. I am not someone who is living the test, but someone who is walking and living in her testimony. You cannot have a testimony without a test.

I own that I was made exactly the way GOD wanted me to be made, and that I am here to help someone understand that living with a chronic condition simply means that you have to grab every opportunity that you can to be happy; every opportunity to try all the things you ever wanted to, and the realization that not everyone is going to understand. It's not your job to ensure that they do. Your steps are already ordered. All you have to do is put one foot in front of the other and stay in motion.

Life was given to us to live and we have to live our best lives. Live it with love, freedom and sincerity. Lisa taught me that I have nothing to defend, nothing to prove nothing to hide and nothing to protect. Amen and Amen.

Possibilities

There is life after a Crohn's Diagnosis and a myriad of surgeries ending with a Colostomy. After numerous major surgeries and procedures there will always be someone who reviewed my history to say "boy God must really have a plan for you there must be something special that you have to do that he keeps bringing you through this." I internalized that message and believed that part of my responsibility is to help others who may be experiencing similar issues after major surgery time and time again I wanted to help them learn to manage their reactions to the diagnosis of 1.

Crohn's Disease; 2. Ostomy; and 3. Body Image. Imagine being a 16 year old at a time in your life when you are planning your sweet sixteen and just starting to date. You go to the hospital for stomach pain and your family gets a death sentence for you. They tell your parents to go home and prepare their papers because you're not going to make it. Imagine how everyone must have felt, your siblings, your friends and then the unthinkable happens they have to do surgery and it is unsuccessful.

It takes Perseverance, Tenacity and Intestinal Fortitude to participate in this journey with Crohn's Disease. This is no easy journey, but no matter what the medical professionals threw at me. I would quietly assure my parents, that I wasn't going anywhere because God had a greater plan to use me to help others.

As a teenager my siblings were always there for me. They came to the hospital daily regardless of how bad I looked. My mother was my prayer Angel she came to see me into every surgery and blessed me and the hands that did the surgery. My father was my advocate and spoke with the doctors constantly documenting all that they told him. It was very difficult for him to watch me go through the various surgeries and pain management.

My schoolmates would come and visit and bring me my homework and tried to convince me not to do it because I didn't have to. But honestly, the homework and the studying allowed me to focus on something other than my TPN liquid diet. You see I wasn't allowed to eat food of any kind for months. I would make deals with the nurses that if they let me have my favorite Dipsy Doodles I would drink my Yoo-hoos that they gave me for nutritional value. And of course I would just chew up the Dipsy Doodles and spit them out because I enjoyed the taste. As a young adult perseverance allowed me to ignore all the things the medical staff told me I could not accomplish. After graduating with my Regents diploma and a general diploma from high school which they felt was phenomenal, I was determined to go to college. The doctors did not want me to attend because they felt that it would be too much stress and tax my system. I compromised with them and told them that if they allowed me to go to college I would stay in New York rather than go away. Still I managed to earn a dual degree from Lehman College. None of this was easy, but nobody said life would be easy. My next step was to take a full-time job in Social Work. Once again they said that this would be too stressful for me and that they did not want me to work yet. I acclimated to my full time job and then enrolled in a Master's Program in Human Services full-time, because time is of the essence. I have no time to waste. I continued working full-time to ensure that I advanced my experience in Administration. I went back to school in 2005 and completed my second Master's; an MSW with a specialization in Child and Family at Fordham University.

As I continue to push myself my husband and children simply shake their heads and call me their hero and continue to support me in whatever I do. They feel like if I can accomplish my goals with my health challenges, they have no excuses not to accomplish their goals. My doctors told me I could not have children, but once again God proved them wrong.

What I Know For Sure

I know that Crohn's Disease is not a death sentence. Many people simply decide it is just too much to manage so they are not going to leave their homes. Well that is certainly one way to deal with it. Believe me I totally understand. I was diagnosed when I was 16. It was quite difficult to understand what was going on, when my doctors didn't even know.

I went into surgery and after surgery I realized that everyone can benefit from an Inspirational Life Coach. We all need someone who can help us to identify and understand where we are and where we want to go. Having a chronic condition can cause us to be delayed in completing our goals. Sometimes it can cause us to stop dreaming because life is a constant nightmare. However, sometimes we have to have tunnel vision keeping our eyes on the prize at all times. We can't allow our circumstances to derail our dreams. I can help you learn how to press pause by altering your thinking instead of a period (believing it cannot happen). We need to keep our dreams alive. Our dreams give us life.

The in-between is what we need to manage. There is so much that life has to offer. The question is: Are you bold enough to grab it? Are you brave enough to live your dream unapologetically?

I can help you identify your goals, look at where you are, consider why you are stuck; and move forward to achieve all that is for you.

Truly being happy is realizing that life is an opportunity; an opportunity that you can choose to take advantage of and mold anyway that you see fit. It's your God given right. Refuse to be held back by limiting beliefs.

Nelson Mandela has a great quote that I live by, "I never lose, I either win or I learn". Who wants to be winners with me? Follow me on Instagram Crohn's Interrupted_llt and like my Facebook page, or tweet me @ArmorerWade. I look forward to hearing from you as we take this journey together. I would love to add you to the Crohn's Interrupted: Living Life Triumph-antly group on Facebook.

What Now: The Feeling That May Come Over You Every Time You Relapse

The amazing thing about having Crohn's is that you never know what to expect next. You can be fine out enjoying yourself one day and totally incapacitated the next. This is very difficult for people to understand. Anyone who has never experienced someone going through these challenges would think that you are making it up; a complete fraud. They may even say to you that they saw you out dancing cutting a rug and can't understand why you can't just go out to dinner; where you don't have much to do.

You may have doctor's consultations and even surgery, thinking that everything will be fine afterwards. Then you continue to have the same or worse experiences time after time after time. The medication didn't work the way that they thought it would. The surgery wasn't as successful as they thought it would be. Your family and loved ones continue to be devastated over and over again. And in the midst of it all you are trying not to show your own devastation because you have to be strong for them, but it is exhausting. Somewhere along the way you forget to feel bad, even when you do. So, how do you handle all of these challenges as they occur when it is not so simple? Like when you have to have an emergency ileostomy following a major surgery because it's the only option to save your life. You breathe; you pray and continue to practice that unwavering, unbreakable faith that allows you to see the other side of this experience.

Now we know that having Crohn's is quite complicated, and nothing is ever simple. But it can be handled by using the old adage of "How do you eat an elephant? One bite at a time."
The best thing about having Crohn's is

having a good team of doctors who really understand the disease and family and friends who are a great support even when they can't quite grasp what is going on. You end up knowing more about your diagnosis than the medical professionals caring for you.

Trauma: Ten Steps from Deaths Door

While attending training for working with adolescents; I had an epiphany as I listened to Dr. Kenneth Ginsburg present on Positive Youth Development. I realized that what I had been experiencing with my diagnosis was trauma.

This led to endless research when I found The National Child Traumatic Stress Network (NCTSN). I learned that trauma can create symptoms and experiences much like PTSD. Repeated trauma puts your emotional, psycho-logical and physical well-being at risk. The mitigation for that risk is you have to build "Community". You have to find a way to connect with people who you've identified as your emphatic and open support. Process your feelings with them. Find ways to discharge energy and intense anger. Going through these challenges can cause you to be resentful. For your well-being you need to nourish your body as best you can. Get as much rest as possible and avoid toxins and toxic people. Breathe deeply.

I am going to share information from the Network that I found very helpful.

**NCTSN relates the following to trauma in cancer patients. I have adapted it to Crohn's patients as these were all critical elements of my experience. (Correspondence, 2016)

Pediatric medical traumatic stress is a set of psychological and physiological responses of children and their families to pain, injury, serious illness, medical procedures, and invasive or frightening treatment experiences.

Stress vs. Trauma
These responses are oftentimes related to subjective experience, vary in intensi-

ty and can be adaptive or may become disruptive to functioning. Many aspects of illness and injury are stressful, painful, difficult to deal with; and strain individual and family coping resources. People try to deal with their ailment without dealing with the trauma engendered by their experience - ranging from extreme fright, horror, shock, extreme pain, life threatening or overwhelm.

There can be a realistic (or subjective) sense of life threats. Medical treatment may be frightening, you may feel helpless, uncertain, or required to make important decisions in great times of distress. Traumatic stress in Crohn's should be considered at the time of diagnosis, at the beginning of painful and difficult procedures; during the ups and downs during the course of treatment; post-treatment; and the threat of reoccurrence and other health concerns. There are several Psycho social interactions that can help one reduce anxiety pain and distress. Chiron-Institute.com helps families to seek support for, and pay attention to the impact of treatment related events. They encourage families to develop strong alliances with healthcare providers. Based on my research with the National Child Traumatic Stress Network, I know my family was traumatized. Research suggests that parents are the key resources for their children's emotional recovery after traumatic injury. My condition was chronic and fluid never really ending. Psychosocial interventions need to focus on individuals and families including siblings. Increase social support, increase coping skills, increase family communication and functioning; and refocus unhelpful beliefs about its meanings and the consequences.

Summary: Pediatric illness and injury experiences are potentially traumatic. Children and parents often feel frightened, helpless, & vulnerable, family functioning is disrupted and coping capacity is challenged;

What Healthcare professionals can do: provide information and basic coping assistance for all children and families; promote early identification and further educate yourself through continuing education, reading professional literature and consultations with knowledgeable colleagues as well as listening to your patients.

What parents can do: you can help your child deal with the frightening illness or injury by gently encouraging your child to talk about it, answering your child's questions if you know the answer or referring them to someone who they can talk to, listening to their concerns, support your child participating in normal activities as much as possible and ask for help if your child's reactions worry you. (National Child Traumatic Stress Network (NCTSN))

I am going to provide you with a brief peek at what trauma looked like for me during my journey with Crohn's. I am limiting my experience here because I do not want to cause secondary trauma.

I remember being 16 and told that I was going to die. Can you imagine how difficult that was for me to process in my undeveloped teenage brain? I was devastated, angry, and then I saw the effects the news had on my family. This was inconceivable; there were so many questions it seemed and no answers. My parents did not have any answers, the doctors did not have any answers and I certainly didn't have any answers. The one thing that we did have though was the power of prayer and faith. We prayed for the right doctors who had the right skills. Eventually after several months they showed up and so the journey went on.

Hearing that I may not make it was said so many times that eventually I became numb to it. Every time some doctor came with the warning, I would tell them "you are not God and he hasn't given me the memo yet, so stop stressing my family out".

Just a few short years ago around Easter

I had pain in my legs and they were very heavy. I began to feel like I could not breathe. I was only able to take very short breaths. I felt like I was having a heart attack. I rushed to the hospital to find that I had a DVT (clot in my leg) and two pulmonary emboli in each lung. Once again I heard, "we have to get you into emergency surgery or you are going to die. Your oxygen levels are too low. We need to put in an IVC filter". An IVC filter sits over your lungs to prevent blood clots from getting into your lungs. This is extremely painful and once it's inserted you have to remain at a 45 degree angle without moving for several hours. My poor family. My girlfriend who was on the way to meet me had to notify my family. They would not even wait to let me give her my pocketbook and she was only one block away. When I came out of surgery I had to witness the panic stricken looks on their faces. I had monitors strapped all over me and all the nurses kept saying was "be still.

You can't move around." It took days before I could complete my required laps around the nurse's station. I had to demonstrate my ability before they would release me. When I was released from the hospital I spent months reporting to the clinic daily before going to work. They had to closely monitor my levels and I refused to stay home.

As life would have it, I was in the hospital recovering from yet another surgery when something went wrong. They wheeled me down for a test and the next thing I knew, they were prepping me for surgery for a lifesaving Ileostomy. My body was so weak, I was sent to ICU.

This is yet another example of what trauma looked like in my life and in my family's life. They were once again told that I might not make it.

I share this with you not for pity or concern, but to inspire you to do more. I want you to recognize that you can handle anything thrown at you. You have to be an active participant. It is way too easy to give in to being a victim, because bad things happen to good people. And I know because this has been an ongoing part of my life. I really force to fit it in around my life and not have these experiences be my life. We can do it together. I can coach you to see the possibilities. You deserve it. (Correspondence, 2016)

Take the Shame Out of Your Game: Coping with Crohn's

Do you know anyone that has to go to the bathroom during the day to have a bowel movement? Do you know anyone who has to go to the bathroom more than twice a day to have a bowel movement? Do you know anyone who has to go to the bathroom at least 6 times a day to have a bowel movement or someone who cannot go at all? Going to the bathroom is one of those taboo subjects societally programmed that most people feel uncomfortable about discussing. Yet, everyone has to do it. One way or another. Having Crohn's you could have to go to the bathroom anywhere between two and ten times a day, or you could be constipated. Not only is it exhausting for you but then you have to deal with all of the comments about the bathroom smelling. Some people complain "why not spray" or "the smell of the spray with the stool is bad" or listening to comments about what's wrong with that person. And I am here to tell you that you are not alone. Everyone who is living must use the bathroom at one time or another to defecate. Nobody's waste smells like petunias. For some reason they seem to forget that when it's someone else that uses the bathroom. But I always say as long as I am not at your desk, in your car or sitting at your dining table when I go to the bathroom then everything should be ok. (LOL) That's what the bathroom is made for. I make sure that when I go to the bathroom I am at the appropriate facility because that is what it is designated to be. I encourage everyone and anyone who has Crohn's to feel comfortable using the bathroom. It is your right. You are as entitled as everyone else is.

It's just a matter that you may have to go more than anyone else and that's okay. I adopted a new motto because Lisa Nichols teaches that we have nothing to hide, nothing to prove and nothing to defend. I refuse to allow the immaturity and societally programmed shame of others to keep me from using the bathroom or trying to find an empty bathroom; because as you know the ladies room is never empty. There are some things that can assist you with this situation though and they are as follows:

1. Sense of Humor; I take it with me everywhere I go and often find myself laughing when I watch people race from the bathroom saying "that wasn't me" when it smells. But what if it was you. Going to the bathroom is a required bodily function if you are alive, and it is a source of relief for those who can after being constipated There are drops that you can put into the toilet before you "Go" or before you empty called Poop Pouri. You can find them on Amazon.

2. There are concentrated sprays that dissipate the smell or eliminate it

all together.

3. Diffusers non-aerosol sprays. I use Scentsy and you can buy an array of products at https://chironsenses.scentsy.us/ the travel tins and sprays are perfect for home and traveling. The diffusers with the oils are also so relaxing.

4. There are various deodorants that you can use if you have an appliance. Adapt or Diamonds are two products which can be used together. If you choose a Scentsy spray you just give two pumps before you empty and two pumps after and voila no smell.

You Can't Have Crohn's Without a Sense of Humor

There are many studies that show humor helps people to live longer and deal with difficult events.

Humor also helps you to manage difficult situations. If you can't laugh at yourself you are taking life too seriously. Even God has a sense of humor. You make plans but God already has your steps ordered. His plan will beat yours every time. Many times I have had to approach my diagnosis with a sense of humor. I refuse to suffer in silence. Laughing has been shown to ease tension, improve your immune system and relieve pain. Laughter produces benefits similar to those derived from physical activity, especially important if your Crohn's has been keeping you from the gym. When we laugh, our blood pressure goes up,

we breathe more quickly and we send more oxygen through our system. "The Crohn's Classroom" (Humor And Resiliency, 2013).
Educating myself and others about a condition that's considered taboo is my passion.

In August 2012, a study entitled "Humor and Resiliency: Towards a Process Model of Coping and Growth" was published in the Journal of Psychology. The study itself was about creating a model to evaluate the effects of humor. There were studies done over the last 20 years that showed how humor can enhance psychological well-being and quality of life, particularly during times of stress. Humor, along with kindness, leadership and love, increased significantly following major traumatic events, such as accidents and illnesses. (Kuiper, 2012)

Another study found a sense of humor to be an important factor in personal resiliency that we call upon to cope with trauma or stress-the characteristic of "bouncing back" in the face of adversity. Laughing and a sense of humor may not be a cure all, but more and more research suggests that laughter can be one of the best coping mechanisms there is. "Crohn's Advocate"

Just recently I was sharing a story about a conversation I had with my sister. It was about who could get out of the bathroom quicker. There are five of us. So I said in my best Oprah voice "I know, you get an Ostomy, You get an Ostomy, you get an Ostomy." We couldn't stop laughing. You had to be there.

Many times I have made the choice to laugh instead of cry. I decided a long time ago that if these Crohn's symptoms were going to keep revisiting me then I would need to find something I could control.

Laughter is a great way to make others feel comfortable when talking about a horrible debilitating disease. I invite you to share with me on my Facebook page

(Crohn's Interrupted: Living Life Triumphantly) your funny stories about how you managed an embarrassing situation.

What Change Can You Affect?

I want to take the shame that people feel out of having Crohn's Disease and all of the symptoms that go along with it. I want to remove the shame around being an Ostomate and all of the overwhelming issues that come along with that. You did not choose this life, it chose you. You have an Ostomy it does not have you. Don't let it become your life; fit it into the one you are living. But you have to keep living, don't give up. You have no idea how strong you really are. Always give your best first to yourself and then to others.

It's important to know that you are not alone. There are others who are having similar experiences and journaling and talking about it to a trusted person pro-vides a great release.

"At some point, you have to make a decision. Boundaries don't keep other people out. They fence you in. Life is messy, that's how we're made. So you can waste your life drawing lines. Or you can live your life crossing them." (Laquanna Chong)

Choosing to Live

On January 8, 2016 I made another decision to live. I limped into the office and half sat down because the pain was unbearable.

My GI doctor sent me to a colleague for a second opinion. Before this doctor who is a renowned GI examined me we sat down and had a discussion. He said that he needed to take my history because he understood from the referring doctor that it was quite extensive. But he wanted to hear my opinion and get an understanding of what I was expecting. This already made me comfortable, because I will not deal with any Doctors who believe their opinion is more important than mine. He assessed me as an individual vs. the cookie cutter approach.

After he examined me, he asked how it

was possible that I was still working and driving myself around the city. He said he simply could not imagine how I was even walking. I told him God's Grace and my will. He wanted to know three things that I wanted to accomplish. Of course I gave four.

I explained as follows:
1. I wanted to feel better and be able to function with pain at a four or five instead of a 12 because giving up wasn't an option.

2. I wanted to be able to continue to get to work and resume taking care of my family.

3. Return to the active lifestyle that allowed me to participate in skating, biking and overall spinning of the world.

4. And I want to continue to impact & encourage individuals that I met in a positive way. And motivate them to continue to fight the Crohn's

Beast.

Well he did say to ask for whatever I wanted. Given my health status and the fact that I had just had surgery November 2015, this sounded unbelievable. He sat and pondered for a while and then responded. He said ok, I can't promise you anything but I am pretty sure that if you have this Ostomy, you will after a time have at least a 60% chance of achieving those four things. This sounded like a no brainer to me. When I spoke about this to my friends and family they had a sense of shock and told me that they would support whatever decision I made.

Some were concerned about body image; others were concerned about how I would manage in my already debilitated state. I bawled my eyes out, said a prayer and moved forward with the surgery. This was to be my second Ostomy, but at least I was involved in this decision. The first one that I had in 2010 was an emergency. This one was planned.

What was to follow I would describe as more life lessons... a gift wrapped in sandpaper. My surgeon told me that the surgery went well. And like all of my surgeries my sisters were right there in recovery when I opened my eyes, and the next day we had a storm of 36 inches of snow. Thank goodness they got out before they were stuck. New York City was shut down and I felt like a Mack truck had rolled over me. I wasn't sure what I was going to do because I did not have the strength, but I had faith. My Sorority Sister Deborah Akinbowale came and spent that weekend with me at the hospital, which was a role that my sisters frequently played. I was comforted by the company and the advocacy. I had to let go and let God and he sent one of his Earth Angels to assist me. She helped me to get on my feet and practice walking so I could get my strength back. My Ostomy nurse came in to give me training on how to care for myself when I was discharged, my surgeon stopped by regularly to encourage me and confirm that everything went well and that I would begin feeling stronger in the next two weeks. I was certainly hoping that he knew what he was talking about and not just giving me a line. I felt horrible. When I was discharged home it was a tough first two weeks home. I had to use a walker to ambulate and thank God I still had it from my previous surgery. I could not get up the stairs without my Sorority Sister and friend Elizabeth on one side and my youngest son Jafari on the other. I had my visiting nurse, physical therapist (PT), occupational therapist (OT) and my wonderful home health aide Liz. Liz is like family to me. I met her 6 years ago and she was so empathic with me that I knew that she was the only one who could care for me this go round. I called her ahead of time to make sure that she would be available to assist me. I knew that I couldn't walk or really do anything for myself. So in addition to recognizing that, I had to act to ensure that I would be up and eating in no time. My older sister Gail asked about my dietary needs and began cooking like there was no tomorrow. My other sister Ayshia was the taste tester and deliverer. She came with giant coolers of food and re-packaged them to give me a great variety. They told me my only job was to eat. This was the best part.

Fortunately, my appetite had returned full force. Everyday my job was to figure out what I wanted for breakfast, lunch and dinner. Because I could digest food differently I began to gain weight onto my tiny frame. I gained a total of 35 lbs. and was just fitting into a small. My husband was always there supporting and working with Liz to get me mobile again. He watched me closely and reminded me to eat and rest. He did not want me to get ahead of myself, which I have been known to do. With each day that passed I got stronger and my nurse, PT and OT kept telling me how well I was dealing with my condition. I kept telling them I don't have a condition just a situation to get through. I told them "I have a diagnosis with some challenges; I have an Ostomy it does not have me. They kept asking me to write a book to help their other patients believe that there was hope. They could not believe that I was planning to return to work in April; they thought it was too soon & I should wait until the summer, but I was having no parts of that. I had places to go, people to see and things to do. I still had many things to accomplish.

She Thought She Could And So She Did; Living with Rosebutt Buttercup

Let me introduce you to Rosebutt Buttercup. She is my new best friend and has had her first birthday on January 20th, 2017. She came along and saved my life, literally. I might not be here if I didn't make the decision to have her accompany me everywhere I go 24/7. Rosebutt Buttercup is the given name of my colostomy. She has a first and last name just like everyone else. I'm ecstatic to have her and I respect her because not only has she given me life but my quality of life has been restored. I wanted to give her a positive name and she has given me so much positivity. I have more than hope now. I have proof. I have gained 40 pounds. I thank God that I feel well. I have energy and I'm looking forward to being able to participate in all that life has to offer me. Rosebutt is my constant companion and I love her. Who knew I would be so happy with a colostomy. I eat better, absorb the nutrients in food better, and I am the fastest one in and out of the bathroom. It might sound crazy but I simply love it. No more running around looking for bathrooms at airports, restaurants, movies or rest stops along the highway. And I want my other Ostomates to give their ostomies a name. There's power in the name. Please Facebook me and let me know what you came up with as a name for yours. I chose a cute positive name because I did not want to create negative energy around my life-giver. Be creative!!

My seven year old nephew saw my stoma and asked "Aunty Mommy what's that on your Power Ranger belt?" I responded "that's my super powers". And to be honest, I feel like it has given me super powers. My friends and family simply ask how Rosebutt is doing. It gives them an easy way to feel comfortable asking about my colostomy. Rose-butt has allowed me to have some very interesting conversations with people. There are 450,000 people who have stomas. There are over a 130,000 people in the United States who have colosto-mies annually. Many are devastated by the procedure and oftentimes do not have the support or supplies or access to supplies that they need. They are not sure how to navigate the system. Deal-ing with any type of Ostomy can be tough and it takes time to get adjusted. Take your time and be kind to yourself, everyone is different. Please know that there are resources out there for you and I am rooting for you. I will share a list of my resources at the end of the book.

It took great courage to move forward with this surgery. I knew what I could handle in regards to pain and managing my life with Crohn's. But I was anxious about having a colostomy because I didn't know what to expect on the other side. I thought I was going to have to wear frumpy clothes to cover it up. But this is not the case. I dress fashionably and you would never know that I had a colostomy unless I told you. Well I am telling. I have worn casual, formal and semi-formal. I will post them on my Instagram Crohn's Interrupted_llt and Makedaarmorerwade.com to give you ideas. The key is the accessories. You can always have a consultation with me, if that will assist you in feeling comfortable.

One morning I had a doctor's appointment and I met a terrific nurse, a beautiful young woman who was very protective of me. She was careful about asking me to disrobe and allowing the doctor to examine me. Normally they ask if you would like a sheet to cover with, but then she began asking are you sure you're going to be okay with the doctor examining you. I told her it was fine and that she could stay in the room if it would make her feel better. I was wondering what the issue was and after we spoke for a time, she disclosed that she also had a colostomy but that no one knew about it.

This visit turned into a dialogue about living with Rosebutt. She was trying to figure things out for herself. I gave up as many resources in the short space of time that I could. I realized that people need support and encouragement around having a colostomy. And while I don't have all the answers, I have figured out what works for me. She was surprised to know that she could still get pregnant and have babies; she wanted to stay in touch. She wanted to know things like how it was to go swimming and go on dates and have relationships. I want to put an unashamed face on having a stoma. Forget the vanity I want to have a great quality of life and you can too. You have to create a circle of people who understand and appreciate that and if you don't have one you can join mine. I want to hear your stories of your journey whether it's you or a family member. How you handled your diagnosis or are currently handling it? Describe what things you see as goals for your future. For example, I am going to love me just the way I am. What are you trying to accomplish? Post to my Fb page Crohn's Interrupted: Living Life Triumphantly.

There is much that I would like to share with you about living with a Colostomy. There were many famous people who had an Ostomy. For example,

Marvin Bush: Son of former US President;

Bob Hope: Entertainer, Comedian, Actor;

Loretta Young: Actress;

Fred Astaire: Actor/Dancer;

Dwight Eisenhower: Former US President;

Ed Sullivan: TV Host;

Tip O'Neil: Former US Speaker of the House;

Queen Elizabeth: Queen of England;

Napoleon Bonaparte: world leader and military conqueror.

I was surprised to find out that so many powerful people had a colostomy. It obviously did not limit them and I refuse to let it limit me. Rosebutt allowed me to see the possibilities, and that led me to become what I call an Inspirational Life Coach.

Traveling

When I decided that I wanted to travel, my family was very anxious. There were six things that I needed to do. And these may help you.

1. Check all of your seals before you board

2. Make sure that you pack your supplies in your carryon bag. If you do not have a precut flange, cut several to carry with you and place the scissors in your checked luggage. They will not let you board with them. If you do not have luggage that will be checked, cut all of your flange's before you travel.

3. Make sure you have twice as many supplies as you think you need.

Never count your supplies exactly. You could be delayed, your bag could get lost; or you may eat something that has you changing frequently. If you go to the pool, beach or sauna your flange may need to be changed.

4. Go to the (UOAA) United Ostomy Association of America and print out the blue card. This can be extremely helpful. It is 2 sided and can be shown to the TSA. You can request a private screening. You do not have to patted down and explain in front of everyone. You can also present it to the stewardess to use the bathroom if the "fasten your seat belt sign" is on.

5. Eat a small meal. I prefer not to eat a huge meal before I am going to fly because then you will have to empty or change your bag. I prefer to do that before and after the flight. But if you are concerned about your bag blowing up, be-

cause you don't have a full stomach; Gas-X works for me. I just
pop one in my mouth after I eat.

6. Travel with your own snacks that
make you feel comfortable. I don't
drink the seltzer beverages offered
because they increase the gas in
my stomach.

Now if you are traveling by car or train or
even bus you may have a little more
flexibility. There were a number of things
that I found helpful.

For instance:
1. When I travel by car I am able to
pack everything that I need however I make sure it is easily acces-
sible.

2. I still make sure that I have
enough supplies to make a quick
change. But there are benefits to
being in your car and not having to
race to a rest stop. Especially at
night.

3. I can burp my bag if I need to and have full control of the venting when needed.

4. I carry non-aerosol concentrated sprays that assist with any pungent smells.

5. I always have a bag over packed with my special items that I can eat. And I identify what is safe to eat on the road just in case I have to stop at a rest area, by doing my research ahead of time.

Enjoy your travels!!!

Tips for Choosing to Live a Productive Life with an Ostomy

I was speaking with someone who was explaining to me that extreme sport athletes who climb mountains and participate in outside sports poop in a bag. This was surprising to me. They said there is no shame with that, as a matter of fact they are champion athletes. We could look at this the same way. Success leaves Clues and you have to look at what has worked in the past and operate from a solution driven perspective. My life has been what Lisa Nichols describes as lessons "gifts" wrapped in sandpaper. Managing my many health issues could be tantamount to climbing Mount Everest. But the old adage applies. You get through one step at a time. I find myself singing the song put one foot in front of the other from the

Christmas movie Rudolph the Red Nosed Reindeer.

I truly believe that it's how you live life and battle through that makes the difference. I am constantly told that I make it sound easy. It is definitely not easy, but my conviction and de-termination keep me grounded. Limiting the complaining is helpful as well. Complaining keeps you in the valley. This disease is already unpredictable and has numerous highs and lows. You have to give your pity party a start and end time. I have one person who is my pity party partner. When needed I pick up the phone, time myself for 15 minutes and go at it. At the end of that time I feel better, it's over and out. Next, and then move on. Having Crohn's can feel like living with the flu and arthritis every day. Many times you are managing daily pain, multiple trips to the bathroom and figuring out what foods you can tolerate. I have been doing well with my meal plan.

I have spent years trying to protect my

loved ones from watching me suffer. So in my mind I chose not to let it get to me. I truly understand how draining, depressing and nerve wracking it can be to watch someone you love deteriorate right before your eyes. I've watched the look on my husband's face and my family when they came to see me in the hospital. I can see the terror and uncertainty when they show up in recovery, surgery after surgery.

So I put my best face on and do my best to convince them that it's not as bad as it seems. But this has been pretty tough. In putting my best foot forward and staying positive, I somehow convinced myself that I am fine. Don't misunderstand; I am not delusional. I still have to make all the medical decisions and coordinate my care but I make sure to do it with Grace and as much control as I can muster. I intend to do it my way, of course following doctor's orders most of the time. But I've been doing my "residency" for a long time and my doctors trust me. One of the things that makes me happiest is teaching doctors about the facets of my condition, knowing this is how it can help someone else. I was once told "you will know more about your diagnosis than most of the medical professionals who will care for you." The severity of my disease always intrigues them. So when I am hospitalized I hold Court. They always have lots of questions and I always have lots of answers, as it pertains to me. For example, I had to explain five times about what Setons are and how they work and why I had them. Everyone wanted to see them and examine me, doctor after doctor after doctor. I told them that they would all have to come back at once and then they can examine me. Setons are similar to drains that are put into an incision to keep it open so that your body can drain and heal. Well guess what, this is not common knowledge even though you would think it is in the medical community. There is so much more that is known about Crohn's Disease now, than there was during my diagnosis and medical journey.

I set simple goals to be met. For instance I concentrated on making it to my kid's track meets and baseball games. Then I concentrated on making it to their graduations. I am looking forward to watching them get married and settle down, & then seeing my grandchildren. If you make constant goals/milestones and focus on them, there is less time to focus on what challenges and issues are happening to you. You establish some-thing to hold onto; something to hold on for. Sometime when I go to the doctor and he asks me how I am doing, I tell him I am not complaining. But he says "no, I need to hear any complaints, we need to address them." This is the type of doctor we all need

Overcome the Fears; The Art of Survival

Overcoming fear is not easy, but if you replace that fear with faith it becomes bearable. I had to believe that things would get better no matter what. I had to believe that with each new drug I tried, that it would solve the problem. Having faith that with each surgery that the solution would be found and the issue would be fixed. With each surgery there was some semblance of improvement but the recovery was always brutal.

There are so many things that people will judge you for. They will never know what has to be overcome just to have a day that they would consider "normal". So worrying about others perceptions is a skill that has to be mastered or it will immobilize you.

As a Crohn's patient and now an Ostomate you have many demons to battle. You have to figure out your daily schedule that includes bathroom accessibility, time to rest due to the fatigue, meditate to relieve the stress and a change of clothes for possible accidents. Always have a plan B, C and D for the rest of it all. Sometimes asking for the help you need is harder than getting the help because you are embarrassed.

Nothing to Hide, Nothing to Protect, Nothing to Defend, Nothing to Prove

Having nothing to hide, protect, defend or prove is the way I have been living my life. But I began living a new life seven years ago. After one of my life saving surgeries, I remember trying to figure out how I was going to get back and forth to my doctor's appointments and eventually go back to work. I was incontinent and constantly looking for a bathroom. So in trying to problem solve and come up with a plan that would allow me to do what I needed to I spoke with my husband. He, being the supportive person that he is, did some preliminary research and asked how I would feel about having a bathroom in my car. I got extremely excited. I would become free and able to travel wherever I wanted.

And most importantly I could get to work and participate in life without using a map to designate places where I could stop and use a bathroom, because we know how unforgiving Crohn's can be. My point is, I try to live a solution driven life. I look at every situation to determine if it's something I can alter or work through. So now instead of trying to figure out the location of a bathroom, I was identifying where I could pull over to use the bathroom without getting a ticket.

That is always fun in NYC. I have had some interesting stops for instance: the Triboro Bridge Plaza, FDR, West Side Highway, NJTP and wherever else I thought it was safe. But you really need to travel with your sense of humor. When I told my hematologist at the I and R clinic (international normalized ratio is used to check whether medicine to prevent clots is working) during my interview how I had been managing since my hospital release, she asked per-mission to share my story. She wanted to share my story with her family at Thanksgiving because she felt her family members were not grateful enough. She could not believe that I would pull over on the bridge or the highway or road to use the bathroom. She wanted to see the set up. I explained that the toilet had a water well and flushed and was quite functional. Being out late trying to find a bathroom just wasn't safe. So this was a necessity. After having two pulmonary emboli (blood clots) in both lungs and DVT (Deep Vein Thrombosis) in my leg diminishing my ability to walk long distances was limited. I would get very winded and feel like I was going to collapse.

Let me share a story that helps to keep me motivated to have a sense of humor. One afternoon at work, at lunch I ate something that did not agree with me. I had a reaction where everything poured out of me. I wasn't lucky enough to make it to the rest room without soiling my clothes. I had a work friend whom I had confided in to get my trusty backup bag that had all the things needed to clean up, change my clothes and return to work. The funny story behind that was my backup clothes were in my car and the car was in the garage and to make matters worse the clothes were too big. I had lost 60 lbs. from the time I bought those clothes to work. I had to get in a cab and go to Dalton's to purchase new clothes. It was the only store in the vicinity. I came back to work changed my clothes and packed up the soiled ones to go home. By the time I did all of that my lunch hour was over and I calmly went back to my desk and started working until quitting time. Now I could have allowed fear of what others may say, force me to go home or isolate myself; but that would break the promise that I made to myself regarding hiding from the challenges of Crohn's. I know some of you may find that embarrassing, but when you have enough of these stories in your life you begin to realize that if you don't laugh about it, you will spend a lot of your time crying. Lesson learned: carry extra clothes to work and make sure that they still fit.

There were so many other times that the reactions of people around me astonished me. And I had to come to understand that because I had to learn how to live with the diagnosis of Crohn's. It didn't mean that the people around me could handle it when they witnessed a bit of what my daily life looked like. I remember being in high school and I just wanted to do what everyone else was doing. So my class went to gym and so did I. I was so excited my restriction was lifted. I was running up and down playing kick ball when my bandage fell off. Being accustomed to irrigating, packing and dressing my own wound twice a day, I figured I could just go to the nurse's office and ask for a new 4x4 bandage. I never thought the nurse would want to see what I wanted it for. So I explained that she might not want to do that and if she just gave me a minute, I would take care of it. Long story short when I showed it to her she almost passed out. She got on the loud speaker and had the Principal and Vice Principal run at top speed to the nurse's office. I was doubled over with laughter trying to understand what the big deal was. They all started fanning themselves wanting to call 911. They put me on the couch with an ice pack on my head and elevated my feet.

There was nothing that I could say that would calm them down, they were calling my parents. I begged please don't do that; just let me redress my wound because the class was almost over and my team was up. They just looked at me. Needless to say they did speak with my father who assured them I could handle it and I did. But they were so scared and traumatized and I understand why this was a big deal. But this is just an example of what I could experience on any given day.

Choosing the Medical Team That's Right for You

1. Look the provider up on the internet to see what others have to say about them.

2. Interview them and evaluate how they feel about you asking them questions.

3. Do they listen to you or do they treat you like the last hundred they treated with a cookie-cutter approach?

4. Do they have time to listen to all of your concerns or are they only interested in the reason for your visit at that time?

5. Do they take your concerns seriously or do they dismiss them?

6. Do they treat you with respect ac-

knowledging your right to speak your mind and be a part of the team and not just a patient who is there for services?

7. Do they have an understanding of Crohn's Disease and understand their Specialty and the need to coordinate care? Will they take the time to speak with you or your other providers who can coordinate your care?

8. Ask your current doctor if they would go to them. Ask around the hospital and certainly speak to the nurses. They always have the real nitty-gritty on what's going on.

9. Does your doctor have a good bedside manner or do they only push their agenda and their prescriptions?

10. Can your doctor smile? Do they smile at you? Pay attention to how they treat their staff are they respectful of them? If they don't treat the staff well, they won't treat you well either.

How to be a Good Patient

1. Research your symptoms and if you have a diagnosis, research that as well. You should make yourself be as well versed as your doctor regarding your condition. Once you do this you will be able to have an intelligent conversation with your doctor.

2. Be a part of the solution. You are a member of the team. Act like it. Do not allow someone else to be in the driver's seat while you ride in the back. Being well-versed about your condition because you studied the map of the terrain will enable you to receive directions and ask good questions regarding the navigation to your destination.

3. Keep a medical journal. You need to

know what medications you have taken and that you are currently taking along with the dosage and time frame. Make sure you check for contraindications and discuss these with your doctor. Read the pamphlet that comes with your medication. They are including it for a reason. If you are in the hospital read every bag of medicine being put up and question everything. Make sure it has your name on it.

4. If you are taking a medication and want to stop it, discuss it with your doctor before doing so. You need to be able to explain the reasons you want to stop it as well as whether it should be replaced with something else.

5. Be consistent. When you have an appointment make sure you keep it and arrive 10 minutes before your appointment time. This allows you to fill out or correct any paperwork that they have for you and then see your doctor on time.

6. Any medications prescribed for you

put them on a track calendar or pill box this will help you to stay on time and hopefully your meds can do their job successfully. Monitor how well you feel with the meds and if there are any changes with your body with their effectiveness so you can report it.

7. Develop a good relationship with your medical team. When you have a good relationship they are better able to understand who you are and can better serve you. They can determine when something is emergent versus just asking questions or looking for information. The responses will be different. When you have trust you can ask anything.

8. Develop a core team. You want doctors who are not only well-versed but who have practiced for a while. Interview them for the job. "You" are the most important part of this equation. Ask around for referrals. Ask the nurses and the doctors in the office who they go to. Look to see if your doctor asks your opinion regarding any referrals that he's made to

you. Give your honest opinion.

9. Don't be afraid to change doctors if you don't feel comfortable or aren't getting your needs met. They are there to serve you. They must have time to answer your questions and you must be prepared to ask them.

10. Always seek clarity and get second and third opinions if necessary. Be sure that you understand your doctor's instructions and if it is something that you don't agree with seek a second opinion; this is why you have a team. You must be able to trust your team! Most of the time I am dealing with life and death. If I am at the doctor, it is something I could not handle at home.

What Not to Do is as Important as What to Do: My Tips for Making it Through the Night without a Rupture

1. Don't eat foods that cause you to have a lot of gas, this includes sodas and other drinks that have seltzer in it. You will have to burp your bag all night.

2. Don't eat foods that will make you active all night such as fried foods. Your intestines need time to rest.

3. Try not to eat too close to bedtime or your intestines will empty all night.

4. Empty your bag right before you go to bed, this way you start off

with an empty bag and you don't have to worry about it filling up so quickly.

5. Sleep on your back or on your side, this will allow you to be able to burp your bag easily while checking to make sure that there is not too much fluid in it.

6. Empty your bag when it's a quarter full, so that if you have to burp your bag the fluid does not come out and it's not too heavy lifting the flange from your body.

7. Sit up or stand to burp your bag so that the contents remain at the bottom.

8. Don't wait for the bag to fill up because it will begin to lift the appliance from your skin and then it will cause your skin to be irritated.

9. Make sure to check for leaks be-

fore you lay down and pretty much every time you use the restroom.

10. Ensure your flange is still adhering to your skin properly and if you find that there is a lot of redness you may want to use stomahesive powder.

Tips for Going Back to Work:
Success Leaves Clues

I have taken the journey of returning to work on so many occasions. When you are making the decision to return to work after surgery there are a number of things that you should consider; because nothing beats a good plan.

1. You need to decide whether or not you are going to share the type of your surgery. Some people find this to be a freeing experience. My decision was to share the information with one person. I did not want anyone to make decisions for me based on my experience. At the time, that is what was comfortable for me. You have to do what

feels right to you. You need to judge your circumstance.

2. Identify at least one person you can trust to share your situation with. I wanted to make sure that if I got into a jam or had a leak I could have someone who would understand and was willing to support me.

3. Determine with your doctors if you need some type of an accommodation. Are you strong enough? Depending on the type of work that you do, you may need an accommodation to be able to handle your daily work responsibility. This would go through your Equal Employment Office (EEO).

4. Determine where you can keep your supplies and a change of clothes. Some

people have lockers and some may have a desk or overhead where they can store additional supplies. This is a good practice. It's better to be prepared and never need it, than to need it and not have those items. Have an emergency set in the car as well if that is applicable.

5. Make sure that you check your seals before and after lunch so that you can enjoy your break.

6. Map out your route to work so that you know for sure where you can stop if the situation arises for you to do so.

7. If you begin to smell your bag, change your appliance as soon as possible. If you are unable to change it, keep surgical tape with you at all

times. It will help you to se-
cure the edges until which
time you can change it.

8. Make sure that you always
have a deodorizer with you
as adults can sometimes be-
have immaturely. I recom-
mend the non-aerosol room
sprays or car bars that can
be found at
**https://chironsenses.scen
tsy.us/**

Consider what type of supplies you need
to have and what is covered by your insurance. Some supplies you may need to
purchase on your own for your comfort.
If something isn't covered, that doesn't
mean you should not have it. You just
have to work it into your budget.

Eat to Live,

Don't Live to Eat

I've been taught to eat to live and not live to eat. Don't get me wrong I love food like the next person maybe even a little more, but had to make some hard decisions. There were many things that were my favorite foods bread, being at the top of the list and then of course macaroni and cheese, fried chicken, curry shrimp, & rice and peas. I love sharp cheddar cheese and ice cream but they quickly became a no no for me.

With every hospitalization I was always told that you should eat what makes you feel good; you should eat the things that make you happy you should eat the things that you can tolerate. When I'm in the hospital that's never an issue because 9 times out of 10 the only thing that I can eat and tolerate are liquids; tea, Jell-O, broth, beef broth, chicken broth and of course lots of water. So any hospitalization I'm definitely going to lose about 10 pounds because I can't have any solid foods. And then when I can have solid foods they start you out slowly with scrambled eggs or boiled eggs and maybe a slice of white bread because that's something that's easy to digest. Most times you are just so happy to be able to eat something you gladly eat it without question. Over the years there were many things that I learned about what I needed to eat and when.

When you identify the foods that are not your friend, you must recognize them as your personal poisons. You have to set yourself up for eating success by coming up with substitutions that work for you and recognizing that like dogs drinking anti-freeze just because it tastes good doesn't mean it isn't harmful. If dogs eat chocolate they can develop diabetes. Identify it as what it is "personal poison" for you and you cannot let it pass your lips. I learned new recipes that allowed me to eat well and bypass my personal poisons. You can do this too!

The hospital will usually have you speak with a Nutritionist. The nutritionist will give you the triangle food pyramid and tell you to eat two foods out of each category of food. They will advise you to try a low fiber diet and then they send you Cream of Wheat and wheat bread for breakfast. Only recently has there been a connection with food and your gut. My nutritionist Dr. Melvyn Grovit identified the benefits of eating in this manner 35 years ago and has been practicing Integrative Nutrition. He has helped me to develop a personalized new way of eating that over time has greatly contributed to my well-being.

Bread was always a favorite comfort food because I felt like it absorbed the acid in my stomach and I never left home without bread or crackers prefera- bly white. Then I was told to eat only wheat bread because that's a healthy choice and of course we all want to be healthy. Thank goodness Dr. Grovit helped me to understand that what is considered to be a healthy choice for the masses was not a healthy choice for me. As a matter of fact, the way that I un- derstand it; when I eat wheat it would go down and form in a ball and cause me to feel bloated. Dr. Grovit had me keep a food journal for a month.

I not only logged the foods but I logged how they made me feel when I ate them. Because remember: I was told to eat what makes you feel good by the hospi- tal nutritionist.

First things first: Elimination Diet, Dr. Grovit had me give up wheat bread, crackers and pasta. I told him that hav- ing me discontinue bread would be like plucking my eyes out. I gave up all dairy; milk, cheese, yogurt and butter. I gave up eating anything that was raw so that included salad foods, fruit and all vegetables. I literally went crazy. I stopped all caffeinated beverages and snacks with high fructose corn syrup and maltodextrin; so no soda, juice, no hot chocolate, no candy and nothing with high fructose corn syrup. I was desperate to figure out what I would be eating. So we started with decaffeinated black tea, lemon and honey, because I wasn't a coffee drinker. Eggland's Best eggs boiled or scrambled, Cream of Rice cereal or Rice Chex with Silk Vanilla Almond Milk and protein to make a shake. Now of course he had me on a special protein that did not have a lot of fillers in them. Believe it or not this was pretty filling and after eating like this for a while your body gets used to it. I even stopped craving those wonderful breads and cheeses and grilled cheese sandwiches with coffee cake or pound cake. The information that assisted me the most was understanding how wheat, yeast and dairy impacts Crohn's Disease. When you test positive for Crohn's Disease it shows an intolerance to yeast. Each of those products causes an auto immune reaction resulting in inflammation. The body erroneously attacks itself trying to protect itself and decrease the inflammation. When you put yeast in bread it causes the bread to rise and double in size. When I eat products with yeast, I feel bloated.

I envisioned looking inside my body and seeing my intestines distended when I ate the wrong thing. My friend at work used to tell me to think of those foods that I should not be eating, as having worms in them. The visual keeps me honest. Eating like this required me to prepare my food ahead of time. I researched different food combinations and hold myself to task to eat right. When I sit with others now to eat, I can only do that if I am going to be mindful. For the first two years of eating like this, I never went into the lunchroom to eat with my colleagues. I ate at my desk. They always had yummy food that would tempt me to eat things that my body would reject. But I've I learned to respect my body. It no longer mattered so much what others were eating. My second big accomplishment around choosing to eat to live was developing my own recipes; I had to learn the hard way that eating gluten free did not mean the contents were soy free, corn free or yeast free.

So here is the good news, you don't have to suffer. There are delicious food alternatives that you can still enjoy. I currently use Silk Vanilla Almond Milk as my milk replacement. I use all different varieties of Tinkyada rice pasta. They have brown and white rice pasta. What I like the most about it is the taste and consistency. It cooks really well al dente and it tastes great. I make all kinds of casseroles, macaroni and cheese and spaghetti meals with it; my lasagna has been just to die for and just so you know I occasionally use the Daiya cheese to replace the dairy cheese. Daiya cheeses come shredded, in slices or blocks. I use Monterey, Cheddar, Smoked Gouda and Jalapeno, I usually grate them. I only use the blocks and the cream cheese because they do not contain inactive yeast.

So I can still put cheese in my omelet or have a grilled cheese sandwich. It melts and stretches pretty well. I cannot use the shredded cheeses because they contain inactive yeast, and I cannot use the Daiya sliced cheese because it contains carrageenan. I have started a personal campaign to get the carrageenan and the inactive yeast removed from their products so that I can enjoy those as well. They have created Greek yogurt in black cherry, peach and strawberry. I use Earth Balance butter. These come in different flavors as well and taste great. I love the butter flavor and the original. I put this in & on just about everything that I make like potatoes, vegetables and I use it to bake my wonderful breads and biscuits. Daiya came out with their own crème cheese, there are three different types. They are plain, strawberry and chives, really delicious on a baked potato. Guess what? It's Dairy free. So far I have tried the plain and the one with chives. They are both delicious.

You can use them to make cheese cake or make a dip to eat with these great organic rice crackers that I found. It gets better, I just recently learned that Daiya now makes cheese cake in several varieties. So if you don't want to make it yourself, there is always Daiya. It does not currently contain anything that I cannot eat. I couldn't believe it but the crackers that I found did not have any of the products on my restriction list either. YOU can find all of these products at Fairway Supermarkets.

I do have a bit of advice about shopping. Always read your food labels to ensure that you are not buying something that you have a food sensitivity to.

Let's talk a little bit about baking. So this was major trial and error and caused me to waste a lot of food. This was difficult for me because I was always taught never to waste food or to throw food out, but once you tasted some of the breads that I first made you wouldn't mind me throwing them away. My first attempts were pretty bad if I have to say so myself. I began using gluten free recipe books for gluten free baking. But the struggle was trying to figure out the substitutions. Because as I expressed earlier even if it's gluten-free it doesn't mean it is corn free, yeast free and dairy free. In other words, I can't eat it.

So after spending a great deal of money on different flours and mixing and measuring them I learned about rice flour from my sister Gail. When I told her that I wanted to experiment she started sending me huge quantities of flour to make goodies to try out. I love bread and my goal was to figure out how I could still have it. Not to mention it would help me to put on some weight. I started out with a sourdough bread it wasn't too bad but it wasn't great either I was trying to replicate the Butter Bread that my mother used to make for us every weekend as children, but this just wasn't working. This is something that I plan to master, because it's a family tradition that I would like to keep and it tastes great. The other recipe that I am practicing now is how to make Roti with this flour. I make things like roast bake and fried bake and these are things that are culturally fun to eat so I did not want to give them up. I love pancakes and waffles on the weekend. So I worked with my sister Ayshia to come up with a recipe that allows me not to miss out on waffles or pancakes. It's a lemon pancake with lemon zest on top. Fantastic.

Fast forward six months. My sister, Gail has always been the champion cook along with her husband, helping me to come up with some great dessert recipes. The following are just a few of the desserts that we came up with. They are Gaily's Biscuits, Mom's butter bread, Jerry's Chocolate Chocolate Chip Cookies, Jerry's Wheat Free Carrot Cake, Jerry's Wheat Free Coconut Cake, and Jerry's Wheat Free Red Velvet Cake. I finally perfected Cinnamon Bread, Banana Bread, Apple Cinnamon Muffins, Honey Biscuits, Pumpkin Bread and Butter

Bread. Based on that information, you can see what my priority was. I desperately wanted to find alternative options for having the foods I wanted to be able to have again. The best part of this is I don't have to cheat now. Did anyone notice that I did not write in detail about lunch or dinner? Well I will provide you a sample of my five day meal plans using most of the items listed above.

And finally, there is a very smooth, sweet creamy ice cream that has the perfect name, "So Delicious". This ice cream works for me and comes in a wide variety of flavors. They have several flavors made with Coconut milk, Cashew milk and Almond Milk. They have Vanilla, Chocolate and Strawberry just to name a few. They have the ice cream bars covered in chocolate, ice cream sandwiches and pint sized containers. So you see with persistence and commitment, you can change your diet and still eat fun foods. They are excellent and the best part of my recovery. I was able to eat them every day in my quest to gain weight. I even introduced them to my friends and they fell in love with them too. The best part of it all is they are dairy free. You can do this!

SUPPLEMENTS have been such an important part of my existence.

I believe that supplements were a major contribution to keeping me alive and have sustained me over time. I had to follow my personalized supplemental guideline closely. I also suffered with malabsorption. "Intestinal malabsorption is when the mucous membrane in the small intestine cannot properly absorb fats and additionally nutrients during digestion. This may cause diarrhea, vomiting, weight loss or lack of weight gain, painful abdominal bloating, irritability, abdominal cramping, anemia, muscle cramping, bone pain and exhaustion."

I took different supplements at various times throughout my life. But if you want to try them you need to do so with proper nutritional guidance. My goal is to be well with diet and supplements, kicking the pharmaceuticals to the side because of the scary side effects. Dr. Melvyn Grovit is a great resource because he has a great deal of experience and has conducted studies at Columbia. He has spoken about the connection of food to the gut for decades and has helped many people to go into remission. He found vitamins in their truest form without a great deal of fillers. Not only that but he prescribes based on your interview which includes assessing your blood work, your diagnosis and your specific issue. He really understands what you are experiencing and he's able to help you to understand the impact of the supplements. I have faithfully followed this guideline.

We have started some and stopped others based on symptoms and recovery. Specific probiotics have helped me immensely with digestion, acid and gas. The Probiotics have been a Godsend. I take it every night before bed and have minimal stomach challenges during the night. I can sleep straight through now.

There are many Medical Doctors who did not believe in the validity of changing my diet and taking supplements to support my health with Crohn's Disease. So when I go to the hospital I always walk with my own stash. I tell them that I have it and I am taking it and they can check with whomever they like. I refuse to have to lie to my providers in order to be able to take what I know helps me. There is emerging evidence that nutritional support directed at inflammatory bowel disease is quite beneficial. It supports that the gut is the first line of defense and you have to add what you lack or cannot absorb. Thanks to Dr. Grovit and my own sister Gail who prepared my food for 3 months post-surgery according to my specifications and limitations. I have happily gained 39 pounds and I and my family are completely ecstatic at my progress. This is the best I have felt in years and I promise you I am enjoying every minute of it. My personal Gastro-enterologist is elated at my progress and I owe much of it to my targeted nutrition protocol. Let me share with you what my food menu looked like.

My daily food menu examples for 5 days

Day One

Breakfast:
½ cup of cream of rice made with water or silk vanilla milk
2 slices of homemade wheat free bread
1 Cup 16 ounces of decaf tea

Lunch:
1 cup of rice (can be white rice or brown rice) white rice is easier to digest
1 handful of string beans
1 small salmon steak
For a snack you can have an apple sauce (check to make sure of no high fructose corn syrup)

Dinner:
1 small sweet potato with broccoli that's steamed well
1 4-ounce steak

Day Two

Breakfast:
2 hard boiled (egg lands) best eggs
2 slices of wheat free yeast free bread
1 cup 16-ounce decaf tea with lemon and honey

Lunch:
½ of a large sweet potato
½ cup of sweet peas
2 small beef ribs
For a snack you may have pears in their own juice

Dinner:
½ white baked potato
1 cup of carrots & broccoli steamed well
1 slice of meatloaf

Day Three

Breakfast:
½ cup cream of rice with cinnamon you

can use water or milk
2 slices of wheat free bread

Lunch:
1 cup rice and peas
½ cup of steamed baby carrots
 with gravy and half a pork chop or whole pork chop if it's not too large
Snack: you may have peaches in their own juice

Dinner
½ a cup of white rice
Steamed baby carrots
 1 baked chicken leg and thigh or bake chicken breast whichever you prefer

Day Four

Breakfast:
2 Scrambled eggs, bacon, home fries
16 oz. tumbler of decaf black tea with lemon and sugar

Lunch:
1 Cup of Tinkyada White Rice pasta w/turkey meat in sauce

½ cup of steamed carrots
Snack
Rice cakes with peanut butter

Dinner:
½ cup of Yellow rice and peas, turkey wings
8oz black decaf iced tea

Day Five

Breakfast:
1 Lemon Waffle (Rice Flour)
2 Scrambled Eggs
1 16 oz. tumbler of decaf black tea w/lemon and honey

Lunch:
½ cup of Rice and beef ribs
16 oz. of water

Dinner:
½ cup of rice with stewed beef & pigeon peas

Snack:
Dole Diced Peaches Fruit Cup

Have 16 ounces of water between meals which will help you to stay away from the sweets and stay hydrated. Avoid drinks that have high fructose corn syrup because they may cause more diarrhea.

Make a point of keeping a food journal don't eliminate documenting anything that you put into your mouth. Track how the food makes you feel when you eat it. Each food has a feeling attached to it. Some foods are comfort foods, and at the hospital I was encouraged to eat what made me feel good and avoid the foods that made me feel ill. So you need to have an understanding of what you are going to have to resolve emotionally if you can no longer have that food item. At any given time you should be able to rattle off the foods that you can and cannot eat, so you know what to pass on. Additionally, you should keep a medical journal. In the journal you should have your medications listed as well as the mg and the amount of times it should be taken.

You should also know the reason that you are taking that prescription, and some of the more common drug interactions and nutrient interactions. Eating light in the evening is great unless you are a night owl. Your body needs time to digest your food before you retire for the night. I tend to have my protein shake in the evening and my heavy meal at lunch time. Makes the digestion at night easier and saves me time with preparation.

Finding Love and Having Children with Crohn's

Finding love and having children was always something that I expected to do. The fact that I was diagnosed with Crohn's was not something that I was going to allow to stop me. So basically whenever I had a date I was always honest up front. I didn't explain every single thing about my diagnosis however I did explain that I had stomach issues. I told my date that sometimes when I ate certain things that did not agree with me, I would have gastric attacks. This was something that most people could understand & accept. Sometimes I would have to excuse myself to go to the bathroom several times in the evening. This sort of became my norm and then it was expected. Sometimes my date would wait patiently for me to get dressed, knowing that I would need to use the restroom before I left the house. Or ask if I wanted to stop at the restroom while they ordered dinner. I think it's important to share your issues and challenges up front. Communication will make a world of difference. And it is always better to be honest. People will either respect that or not.

But it gives them the opportunity to decide if this is something that they want to deal with. We don't have a choice. Wherever we go, there we are. The worst thing that you can do is have someone become invested and then tell them. I know that a lot of people are scared or uncomfortable about letting others find out about their challenges, because they are afraid to be judged. And I know that this can be difficult and sometimes it has been difficult for me. But I always say you feel the fear and do it anyway. Most of the time it worked out just fine for me. I found the man of my dreams, the love of my life, a man who made sure he brought romance to my life. He loves, accepts and respects me, even though I vomited on his shoes. Thank God he has a great sense of humor. We have been together for over 25 years and have three wonderful sons. I could not ask for a more supportive relationship. Occasionally you get someone who did not sign on for that and it allows them to be honest and make the best decision for them which ultimately becomes the best decision for you. This way you don't have to worry about what may come up later on. And you both have options. I love options and believe that is the only way to go.

When you have identified the right one, there needs to be continuous open dialogue about your condition and set clear expectations.

Consider the following:
1. Be honest about what you feel you can contribute or share.

2. Make a plan regarding the activities you are able to participate in

and explore the one's your partner has identified. Maybe it's something you haven't thought about.

3. Determine if you want to have children and/or if you already have children create a plan of action. You will need to know who will handle the children's schedules and how the household is going to run when you are not able. How will the responsibilities be met? How will your family function without your assistance?

4. Create a living will. A living will details your desires regarding your medical treatment in the event you are no longer able to express your desires and consent, especially an advanced directive.

Family and Friends- Give Their Impressions and Perspective on What it's Like Having a Friend/Family Member with Crohn's Disease.

Mom (Dr. Audra Armorer)

My experience as a parent of a child with Crohn's Disease is a very daunting and harrowing one. I have one of the most resilient, persistent, spirited, tenacious, determined, daughter's in the world. To say that I am proud to be her mother is just a fraction of how I feel. My child has managed to battle this tragic disease with determination and Grace. We had been back and forth to the doctor many times before we ever heard the diagnosis of Crohn's Disease. When she went for her first surgery they cancelled it because she went from excruciating pain to no pain at all. Instead of doing a test to find out why, they were relieved, treated her with antibiotics and sent her home. They kept her on antibiotics for 6 months but she still had pain and fever. Eventually we found out her appendix had ruptured hence the release of severe pain. Thank God for our dentist because he referred us to his brother who was a general practitioner who did not like what he saw. He referred us to a friend who was a surgeon and he was the one that saved my daughter's life. We had many sleepless and scary nights not knowing if she was going to make it and I had other children to care for. My husband and I were nervous wrecks. We just didn't know how we were going to get through this thing.

Flare ups every so many months. There are so many stories that I can think of that would give me or anyone pause. But she just works it in stride. It's almost like she just adds it to her schedule like something else to do. I have watched my child suffer for so long before she got the diagnosis of Crohn's Disease. It scared me to death when she had her first major surgery that got infected. They had to hospitalize her in quarantine to protect her from any additional infections. She was a mere 78 pounds and they had to feed her through a tube that went into a vein in her neck called a TPN.

Every time I went to see her I had to put on a gown, a mask and the brightest smile that I could muster; but it broke my heart. She would be sitting there doing her studies and preparing for her Regents exams, because she was determined to take and pass them to obtain her Regents Diploma.

When they finally decided to release her it was because she had convinced them that she could irrigate and pack her own open wound to force it to heal from the inside out. I could not imagine how she was going to handle that because I could not even look at it. The child had a 4 x 3 x 2 open wound on her lower stomach. But she woke every day to irrigate and dress her wound so that she could go to school. She was weak and had to walk with a cane because the ligaments between her knees shrunk. But she was determined to get back to school. What was amazing to me was she never tried to use her illness as an excuse or for any type of gains. Most kids would jump at the chance to stay home but not my Makeda. I would watch her leave extra early in the morning because it took her longer to walk to the bus stop. Then after reaching the school bus stop she would walk three long blocks uphill on Bedford Park Boulevard to get to her school which some describe as a mountain.

One day she was feeling pretty good and decided to go to gym to play with the other students. Her bandage fell off and she went to the nurse's station to get another. The nurse of course wanted to know why she needed gauze pads and tape. When Makeda showed her the open wound she got hysterical. She notified the Principal on the loudspeaker and told

my husband to come to the school immediately. He ran right over to meet a
very nonchalant child explaining that all
she needed was gauze and tape. She
tried to reassure them but they would
not listen.

From this day forward Makeda was put
on restriction to use the elevator, no
gym & given extra books to leave at
home so she wouldn't have to carry
them. They were flabbergasted that she
hadn't asked them for help but that's my
child, she just pushes through. Operation
after operation after operation, it was
grueling exhausting & just too many to
keep count. I just never know what to
expect, the disease is so unpredictable.
One minute she looks fine and the next
we are going back to the hospital for
surgery or a test or new medication. This
would have been easier to deal with if
there was more information at the time.
That's why I am happy Makeda decided
to write this book. I believe that people
would be able to handle the situation
better if someone could tell them what to

expect or give them an idea of what it could be like or even where they could find support. I wish we had someone to speak with.

When the doctors wanted her to wait to start college she told them absolutely not. "I can be home sick or I can go to school sick, but time is going to pass either way and I am going to make the best of my life. If I check out of here I'm going out on my own terms." Not only did she complete College in four years but she did a dual degree with an internship and had the nerve to get a job on top of that.

When she graduated she began working as a Social Worker and went back to school to get her Master's Degree. In the midst of all of this she was still having numerous surgeries, caring for children and family and pushing through. She continues to mesmerize her doctors who love her resilience and positive outlook. They often tell her they wish she could speak with some of their other patients to offer encouragement. So she has taken them up on that.

In 2005 she graduated with her Master's degree in Social Work from Fordham University while working full time. She never ceases to amaze me. Brilliant and always so full of life. And then tragedy hit once again; she had two major surgeries back to back within a week of each other. We thought for sure we lost her this time. After the first surgery the incision did not seem to be healing properly. So they had to do an emergency ileostomy. We found out that she had sepsis and the Doctors were fearful as well. She came out of surgery and was in ICU for over two weeks. She was so swollen that she was unrecognizable. I never knew a head could swell so large. Her eyes looked like they were coming out of her head, but she had a great big smile on her face. She tried greeting us but she couldn't talk and I couldn't watch her like that, I had to run from the room. I felt like screaming. There were about 12 young people waiting to see her and they kept saying that she was their mother because that's the only way they could get in to see her. She really does have that many children even though she didn't birth them. That loving caring spirit of hers just makes you want to be in her presence. They would only give us 15 minutes at a time and she was basically out of it so we each stole a few moments and hung out around her as much as they allowed. I needed to see my child but I could not go often. It was just too much to absorb. Her husband, friends, children and other family kept vigil. I am a faithful praying woman but again I questioned God if she was going to make it. Fast forward four weeks. I was happy when they were able to send her to rehab. But that's when the real recovery without the medical team began. I watched her learn to walk again and fight to eat her meals. The ileostomy was quite an adjustment.

One day I took her to the doctor for some follow up test and her pressure was so low that they said she had to be admitted to Ambulatory Surgery, where they could give her lots of fluids because she refused to go to the ER. The more fluids they gave her to hydrate her is the faster it poured out of the ileostomy. She handled it like a champ trying to comfort me, but I was having a fit and had to keep leaving the room. The one thing that kept me sane, was knowing that they were going to reverse the Ostomy and she told me to just do a countdown. YOU have no idea how difficult it was for me to continue to watch this. It aged me, the constant worry. My daughter kept reassuring me and her sisters. It got to the point where we would have to physically see her because she would not complain. She just kept saying she was fine and on the phone you could not tell. All she talked about was getting back to work. Her medical team kept telling her that she needed time to heal. Her nurses, physical and occupational therapists had their hands full trying to convince her she wasn't ready for certain activities yet. She was on a walker for Pete's sake.

Finally the day came for them to do the reversal of the Ostomy and we thought ok all is well and she can go back to work. But not so fast. It took a few months for her to build up her strength. Finally she was able to go back to work. She was moving slowly but she was going. Fast forward four years and my child is back having yet another major surgery. This time she had a Colostomy. With this surgery again we had high hopes because I had watched her unbeknownst to her coming in from work daily; so exhausted she could not climb the stairs. She would sit and work up the courage and energy to climb the stairs. And each day she would repeat the process. It would just break my heart.

Now 6 months later, she is doing great. She has gained 39lbs. on her special diet and is involved in everything going on. She is truly enjoying life and looking forward to helping others with this disease. She has been giving talks on ostomies with lots of encouragement and tips for balancing life. She's living her normal life and thank God for the doctors that have worked on her. It's a shame that her father did not have the privilege of seeing her actually in remission of Crohn's because he died from an accident; but your mother and family continue to pray and root for you. You are our hero!

Jeffrey Wade (Husband)

I have been so devastated by my (wife's) hero's experiences that I can't even put it into words. She is my everything and I am just thankful that God has allowed her to continue to be a vital part of our lives. I am grateful that she is still with us. She is a wonderful wife and a fantastic mother. We are blessed to have her.

Jason Wade

When I found out you were sick, I was really hurt. It hurt me more when I saw you bounce back and go back to work, get sick again, go back to work. Taking care of the family without missing a beat. Wow... wish I could have helped more at that time. I didn't really understand what was happening. You never really spoke about your diagnosis. You simply told us you were having some challenges and it would be ok. You made it ok for us to go about our daily tasks without too much worry. But when I came home and saw how tiny you were it really blew my mind. I couldn't understand how you took things in stride and kept on moving. Sometimes when I don't feel well, I think about you and just get up and get dressed. The crazy thing is you never stop taking care of the family. Just like "Wonder Woman". You are always in my prayers and I know God has his hands on your life. You are an inspiration to me.

Jafari Wade

For as long as I can remember my mom has had Crohn's disease. I never really knew that's what it was because she was a champ at making me think she was alright. She never wanted to cause me to worry, so she minimalized her challenges well. When I was very little there were times when my mom would disappear. I had my grandmother and my dad who would take care of me when she was gone. She always told me that my job was to focus on school and get good grades and everything else would be okay. But let me tell you what I really experienced from my perspective of course......When I turned 13, I remember my mom going into the hospital. I was worried, but she kept the focus on me.

I always wanted to make my mother proud of me no matter what. I would study and try my best to overcome whatever fear I had on my own. I knew this would make her smile. Even though I had my dad and grandmother, there is nothing like a mother's love and understanding. When I saw my mom disappear for different periods of time when I was little, I knew that meant she was in the hospital. But when she was well, my mom would attend all of my sport activities and mother the other kids on the team who were there as well. As I got older I would just keep trying to focus and keep my grades above a 3.5 average. When I turned 15 I turned up my efforts, working during the summer as a janitor and doing my chores at home.

My mother came to my school and joined the PTA to work as VP and President with my Principal. She made sure that I and everybody else had what they needed to succeed. My Principal and all the teachers loved her. This was no easy task for me to live with, because she held the bar high and my teachers knew this. And then I found out my mom had relapsed again. In my mind I thought that everything was on me now. I had to step it up and be a man for my mom and dad. I did my part to keep the house and my family together. No one knew the pain that I felt as I walked, day by day to school and came back. I had to deal with school teachers that told me that I would not make it to college. I had my friends that were not doing well in school and some ended up dying shortly thereafter. And I had my mom constantly telling me that it would be okay. To overcome this I had to have tunnel vision and exercise that faith, that my mom seemed to have. I believed that God would help me to overcome and bring my mom back to me. When I turned 17 I graduated Aerospace High School in the top 7 of my class and I was heading to college.

I thought that my road will get harder but I learned to be strong from my parents. My mom finally came home but still struggled quite a bit. I played a man as best I could, until I saw that I was a man. When I turned 19 my mom was going through different Naturopathic treatments to improve her health. She was always our champion, encouraging us to do well. My mom in my eyes was the strongest most determined person I have ever seen. She was always thinking of me even when I was thinking of her. She helped me to prepare to attend college.

She loved me & she cared for me. She made sure I was number one even though I wanted her to be number one with all of her health challenges. She showed me I was number one. I don't know any other person that had to fight for their life like my mother. My mother fought for a decade to just feel normal. She taught me to respect life and to respect other people's life. I learned to become a man and to take care of business in the best way. This year, now I am about to graduate College Magna Cum Laude and I see

my mother feeling better and I thank
God every day that my mom is with me.
My mother is a blessing and I love her.
She shows me that we have to respect
life and love it. We have to take advantage of life every day because tomorrow is not promised to us.
We have to always do our best and share
the love that we feel towards each other.
I'm glad that I'm able to tell my mother I
love her every day. I'm glad to make her
food and to do whatever she asks of me.
I want her to feel loved and to feel wanted every day. God is the best and this
family is blessed.

Dorothy Dorsey
Makeda Armorer-Wade is:
A woman of joy, love, peace and beauty;
A woman of intellect, class and distinc-
tion; A woman of knowledge, humility
and tolerance; A lady of wealth, wisdom
and sophistication; A lady who is innova-

tive, self-reliant and responsible;
Makeda Armorer-Wade is one who balances exceptionally well the responsibilities of a devoted wife;
Of a dedicated mother; Of an excellent employee; Of a Dependable daughter and sister; One who manages extended family demands, personal and professional relationships; and organizational affiliations successfully; One who extends herself without reservation sometimes serving as a caretaker, assisting seniors whenever and wherever the need arises; Being a responsible, reliable neighbor; Maintaining a safe, healthy, clean environment for her family;
Makeda Armorer-Wade is a person sensitive to the needs, feelings and desire of others;
A person who multitasks to serve family, work, and organizations without thought;
 A person who reaches out to assist/ satisfy others without consideration of her

own needs first; A person whose endurance for pain floors the average person; A person who after innumerable surgeries, her enthusiasm and zest for life exhibits amazing hope as she fights to encourage others to feel and live that same hope like a beacon of light; A person who takes what life issues to her after critically examining the options, explores other resolutions/theories improvises to meet her needs/ others, or create more alternatives;

Makeda Armorer-Wade is an amazing, concerned, attentive, caring, incredible, pro-found, gifted, honorable, human being. One who makes a difference in the lives which she touches. One of endurance, power, brilliance and spirituality.

A woman of strength and calculation; A woman who bears well with suffering... physical, emotional, & mental, never neglecting/fulfilling her responsibilities.

 A woman who does in-depth research on

diagnosis, medical practices and resolution in relation to her health;

A woman in action exhibiting Supernatural powers in overcoming the medical challenges that attempt to interrupt her style of living and dress; What can we say? She is just super.

A woman of courage and self-motivation who reaches out to encourage/influence others to keep the faith through trials and tribulations.

A woman whose heightened optimism demands a sincere desire from those medically challenged to succeed with assurance that all is well.

Michael Armorer

When I first heard of your illness, I was concerned, but outwardly you still seemed fine so I was not overly concerned. I felt like I had some understanding of what you were going through. Concern for how your life had/would be changed, anger that this had happened to you and frustration because I didn't feel there was anything I could do to help. However, as time progressed, through seeing you, talking to you and others it became clear that your condition was deteriorating significantly. It was at this point that I began to experience feelings of sadness, guilt, frustration and anger. You had lost a lot of weight and were in considerable pain almost constantly. Although, I had some understanding of what you were going through; I had a variety of feelings regarding what you were going through.

Initially, I was sad that you had this illness and I was hoping that there were treatment options that would be the cure. As time went on and I learned more, I was sad that you were dealing with such a serious illness that had such a significant impact on your life. Somehow you managed to handle this madness with such Grace. The impact on me was I thought of you frequently, wondering how you were feeling but not wanting to intrude on your privacy. I tried to cope getting information from you, by educating myself and letting you know I was concerned for you and willing to support however I could.

It might sound kind of strange but eventually I progressed to feeling guilty because I felt like here I am healthy and you are dealing with a debilitating illness and did nothing to deserve it. I felt frustrated, because I was not near you and I felt there was nothing I could do directly to make your situation better. Lastly, I felt anger; not understanding why this had happened to you and why there weren't any cures available.

My immediate response was thinking what can I do? Guess that's just the problem solver in me. I started researching your condition so that I could understand it better and have a greater appreciation for what you are experiencing. I called/texted you just to check in with you to see how you were. I know that sometimes you were not feeling well so I tried not to keep you on the phone too long. When we did talk I tried to be a good listener and offer whatever thoughts I had that might be relevant.

I did find it helpful sometime to talk with other family members about how you were doing (you know sometime you didn't want to give the **real** story). In addition, when it came to you making the decision to have a colostomy, I was comforted by the fact that you had a positive attitude about your decision. I knew that you had researched your options thoroughly and were at peace with your decision. That helped make it easier for me to be positive as well. So glad you are doing much better now!

Beverly Armorer

My perception was my little sister's life was failing fast and I couldn't find the appropriate assistance. I didn't understand everything that was going on. I thought I was going to lose my sister and my friend. It was and still is a very emotional period. Myself and nuclear family wished and prayed for her health to improve. I called more to talk about nonsense and keep up lil' sister's spirits. It was very depressing to watch your sister go from vibrant and energetic to a depressive and withdrawn person.

Makeda's illness has been an emotional weight on my heart. I lost my bubbly sister, the happy one, keeper of the family's jokes!

She was the life of all family events. Then one day she was gone, happiness turned from joy to sadness and gloom. It was a time of depression for me. I lost my sister friend whom assisted me with and shared life experience and rearing of our children together. I woke up one day & life had completely changed. I couldn't cook her favorite food to get her to smile. At family gatherings she rarely ate anything and looked unhealthy. All family gatherings she attended were tailored to her needs. None of the family wanted her to feel left outside of any activities.

One weekend we wanted a sisters' weekend and we rented an apartment in Brooklyn to remain in contact with her doctor. We went out to eat but it really hurt to know she could not eat and there was a withdrawn painful look on her face instead of laughter. We could no longer discuss nonsense on the phone for hours. She did not have the energy or the tolerance. I gave her a gift of time just to see her smile. She said thank you but never shared her smile.

The illness is devastating to the family as every part of life must be re- evaluated.

No matter how you feel you plaster a smile on your face and make the day brighter. I love her to pieces and she appears somewhat better but I am fearful because you never know how long she will be standing.

Gail Armorer
My little sister has been intrepid since she was a tiny baby. Whenever there was a climbable surface she climbed it. She was always reaching for the top of everything. Up! Up! Up! was always where she could be found reaching the tops of appliances, cabinets, closets. She was always engaged in doing things that seemed impossible walking over the ridgepole of the swings at the park, dancing on the top of the monkey bars. That was my baby sister. So when she became ill, she became a shadow of her former self, she couldn't walk, wasn't allowed to eat for months, and was so unhappy I could feel her misery viscerally and it seemed unending! I was so frustrated that I couldn't help her shake this beast named Crohn's. I remember her

being so ill that I would drive 100 miles from where I lived to spend the evening in the hospital and drive back home to go to work for weeks. If Crohn's was a person I would have killed it with my bare hands for all the pain it put her through, but there was no target to conquer except helping her however I could. I was truly happy when she asked me to cook for her and prepared months of meals for her household. I got to work with her dietary limitations to prepare delicious and nourishing meals that brought her from 89 pounds to her current vibrant weight. She has been a trooper through this entire experience and continues to manifest the spirit of Up! Up! Up! In every aspect of her life.

Ayshia Armorer

Makeda, I have a lot of memories around your Crohn's diagnosis. Here are a few:
I remember feeling sorry for you that Thanksgiving Day when your tummy hurt so much that you laid on the sofa for hours not talking. That was such a departure from your usual vibrant counte-

nance. Anyone who knows you, knows you don't lay around in silence! You went to the hospital that next day and came back with no pain, I thought they were miracle workers only to find out later that they were lazy and didn't discover your ruptured appendix. That poison damaged your insides and your life was never the same. I witnessed our dad cry! This was not his style. You came home from the hospital after one of the surgeries with an open incision that had to be debrided, irrigated and not allowed to heal because the infection had to have a way out of your body. That left an incredible scar. You took it all in stride and took over the job as soon as you could, not to have to look at the pain in your parents' faces.

We watched this scene repeat over and over as each Crohn's flare robbed you of inches and inches and feet of intestines and vitality.

I remember struggling to keep up with my studies because I kept running back to New York (the doctors did not expect you to live) I never prayed that hard for anything and I did not want you to die feeling that your sister did not consider you important enough to show up. You were seventy something pounds just eyes and teeth. It was scary.

We knew when you were starting to feel better when your mouth came alive the tongue was and still is mighty! LOL! You would give it to us with both barrels. I thought it was pretty funny, most of the time. Others didn't always see it that way.

I wish it ended there, but the cycle of flare- infection- pain - surgery partial re-covery- and more pain would be repeat-ed over and over again. You had steroids that literally inflated you and hurt your joints. You bought a folding cane and kept it moving! I stopped counting around the 17th surgery It was easier to be ignorant. But I admire your tenacity and willingness to fight. I believe that to be your biggest strength. Your empathy and willingness to help others deal with their health when you weren't well yourself is admirable.

Your diminished health took a terrible toll on our mother and it was hard to witness her witness your pain. She would watch you come home from work and pull your car in the driveway. She would be on the telephone with me and describe how it took 20 minutes for you to get out of the car in slow motion and another 10 minutes to climb 1 flight of stairs to your front door. I cannot fathom how you drove a car and sat at work all day on the Setons.

The pained expression on your face used to make her cry. I couldn't be there, but would offer comfort on the phone. I would give you a chance to get in and settled and call your phone. You never let on that you were having a hard time until it was catastrophic!

Don't ask me how it happened, but in between the cycles you managed to snatch a life. You went to college, you got multiple degrees, you were gainfully employed, you got married, you had children, and parented other's children, and you volunteer and have a rich social life.

I can only say that you demonstrate every day that your attitude determines your altitude. I always wonder what else you would have done if Crohn's didn't keep derailing you. You would just keep starting over. I remember this one time when you had to have a blood transfusion. We were all worried and excited trying to figure out who could get you there and bring you home. YOU took it out of our hands. When we asked how you were getting there and who was going with you. You laughed and said I am taking myself. You never saw any of this as a big deal and I have so much respect for your understanding of how we felt and shielding us from what was going on to calm us.

Your crazy sense of humor is delightful.

You tend to de-escalate crises and bring a calm to situations that would otherwise be utter chaos. You are an example of the way to take life one day at a time and worry about tomorrow- tomorrow. That didn't mean you didn't plan and orchestrate us to distraction but we love having you with us and I personally couldn't imagine my life without you.

...so there, you have me crying at lunch...

My Little Big Sister: Dr. Sharifa Armorer

Life with my little big sister, and oh what a life it is. We spent countless hours together playing and fighting. We were closest in age but she is older than me.

I've always had several sisters some older but this particular sister closest in age and older than me but due to her circumstances she's younger than me. Many times as we were growing up I would be doing the things that a big sister would generally do for a little sister. She had become very ill when I was 10 years old and I remember being very helpless as to what was happening with her. I didn't quite understand what was going on and when they finally diagnosed her it was something we all questioned. At the time they said it wasn't a disease many people of color had. We had a normal life; we played, we read books and enjoyed each other before she became so ill. I thought I was going to lose my sister. So many things changed as she was in high school. We went to the same high school, but I was years behind her. It was difficult living up to the larger than life memories of her great determination as a student.

I took a backseat and watched her struggle as a child. I became her big sis always taking care of her but fighting with her nevertheless. Time progressed and we learned how to deal with her many health issues. My parents would not burden us, but instead tried to shield me from their sadness. My dad was not one to show a whole lot of emotion however he cried many nights wondering if he would be burying his daughter. She is a very strong person. She has weathered many storms and I was right by her side for most of it. As I got older, most times I went to the hospital to see her and to be her advocate, taking care of her while letting them know she has a pit-bull on a very short leash. I recall her having many surgeries and I was often there attending to her needs. I remember the summer of 2011. For some reason she was severely dehydrated. They did not want to discharge her from the hospital because she needed to stay on IV fluids. Makeda being Makeda, convinced the doctor's to let her go home. She did not want to stay in the hospital for the summer. She had them put in a port and have someone train her to give herself her IV's. I was trained as her backup, but I never needed to back her up. She gave herself those IV's every 8 hours. It amazed me to watch her in action.

She did what she said she would, and says what she is going to do and that's just the facts. Makeda is the reason that I returned to school and became a naturopathic doctor. I would treat her with my crystals and other natural healing tools. I created a protocol just for Crohn's and her in particular. And while we don't have any scientific studies her body began to assimilate the nutrients greatly improving her health. We were able to minimize her pain until it is now non-existent. In addition, I also became a surrogate to her sons who affectionately calls me Auntie Mommy. I would attend school functions and support them with her husband. We have a very strong family who will be there when needed to rally around to make a way, where there is no way. We'll help each other mentally, physically, emotionally, spiritually and financially. I love my little big sister and don't plan to be without her.

I am thankful that she has been making improvements, is able to dance and cook and be Auntie Mommy to my son. She has come a long way and can attend events and conferences without restrictions and pain. I am just thankful to God that he has given her a new lease on life, put a smile back on her face, has lifted her spirits in a way for her to be able to deal with all aspects of life, work, home and most importantly her own wellbeing. I know that her message is going to reach far and wide. She has a way of inspiring and helping others see through their challenges regardless of what they are.

Elizabeth Abel

Makeda Armorer-Wade is my line sister and has shown me what it means to be and have a sister. She and I have spent many hours together enjoying each other's company and experiencing life's journeys. Once I learned of Makeda's diagnosis with Crohn's Disease, I wanted to learn more. The best way I understood it was that certain food basically was poison to her intestines. I watched her battle this disease with such Grace and poise, while I thought she was losing. Any and every day could be filled with bathroom runs, changes of clothing, hospital visits, infusions for dehydration and iron, (I think), just to make sure she can get through a day of work. The portable toilet in the car (because she just didn't want to be caught out there), surgeries and significant changes in her weight depending on which meds she was on might have ultimately taken more a toll on us watching her deal with all of this. She always maintained such

Grace and determination to live. Her disposition for life was and is infectious. She never gave up at anything and she often has had more information than the doctors did with new and alternative ways for healing, health, and surviving.

Makeda is simply amazing. I am so happy that she allowed me to be a part of her journey. We have so many stories where the bathroom and hospital visits are involved. I am thrilled that with this last surgery she has been able to truly live again. She is an active participant in her own life and not just sitting by and watching as everyone else around her lived theirs. She truly is a super woman, defying the odds of what she was told she would never be able to do. She is a role model for anyone who has to deal with this Disease and for every person she comes into contact with. This is why we dubbed her The Blessed Phoenix. With God's Grace, she just continues to rise from the ashes.

Liz Flores

I met Makeda over 6 years ago on a semi brisk day, I waited for the door to open (now knowing her, it should have been Jeff, Makeda's husband at the door. She was on bed rest. But a woman walking slowly with a rather larger than life smile answered. I was to be her Home Health Aide. But to my surprise she became my mentor whom my life would not have been the same without.

Makeda's Tenacity and Perseverance is one I attempt to live up to. I paid close attention to her outlook on life, only positive words and affirmations as well as positive words of encouragement ever exited with truths of course of how you might not be living up to your potential. She saw the best in those who crossed her path.

I looked at her and although she had health issues that plagued her, you would have never ever known it. Makeda had just a hiccup of a health issue if you ever asked her. If you asked her how she was doing, somehow the topic ended on you and if you didn't pay attention the focus was now on You! I worked only two days a week 2-3 hours, but our conversations meant the world to me. And along the way the line of HHA/Patient that line was crossed Makeda was an extension of family. A positive role model I wanted to imitate. The Educated Black women, AKA Sorority Gal, Super fun yet realistic Mom who expected her children to excel, the fun Loving Wife, Friend and Family member who you want in your corner. In my mind I created excuses for why I personally couldn't accomplish every-thing, but here we have a women who has faced sickness in the midst of Life and still she made time and sacrifice for all that she has achieved. We, including myself tell her to slow down but, is this really possible? When a simple thought or event is given 300% by this petite extraordinary women named Makeda Armorer Wade.

We conversed one day as I made her king size bed. Although for some it's an easy task, at the time it was hard for her but she still tried and this strong women whom I considered Larger than life in her frail petite self was accustomed to being demanding and in control.... I still had to tell her over and over again stop it! This is my job and her job in my presence was to relax. What a hard task for Make-da!!!!! Mostly the conversations focused on me and her funny stories of her Family, rarely was it focused on her. What I gather from our time was the woman whom she was....but she was still that woman but the angle was now different. Each time I went to her house I learned more about her but in the process I learned more about my-self. And I would like to think I was definitely a part of her recovery in the renewed Makeda Armorer Wade. The physically hands on Makeda was now replaced by a still physically hands on Makeda but with limitations. Let's be realistic who is really going to tell Makeda what she can or can't do. We can only Try!

Now a lot of this will sound repetitive but

I learned so much and Makeda asked me one day what were my long term goals were and I had none. I was living in the world, with no real purpose. Makeda had a gift of showing you; just how to find your purpose by simply asking a question How was this possible? She implanted these tiny thoughts and watered them and she watched them grow. Her Influence on this world is a mustard seed of Faith.

And I am fortunate to have the opportunity to know her and care for her.

Simone Lowry (Symi)

One day my doctor informed me that I have PCOS, <u>Polycystic ovary syndrome</u> ("pah-lee-SIS-tik OH-vuh-ree SIN-drohm"). This a problem in which a woman's hormones are out of balance. It can cause problems with your menstrual cycle and make it difficult to get pregnant. The body may have a problem using insulin, called insulin resistance. When the body doesn't use insulin well, blood sugar levels go up. Over time, this increases your chance of getting diabetes.

It was as if the doctor had given me a life sentence. The questions swarmed my head as the uncertainty of my future became questionable. Will I have difficulty getting pregnant? Will I ever be able to have kids? Who will want to marry me knowing this? It was as if the doctor had given me a life sentence. I'm not a diabetic but have to eat like one? How do I do that?

Watching Makeda deal with Crohn's Disease made me ashamed to even complain of my own situation. She prepares her meals regardless of fatigue. She alters her meal if it has ingredients she cannot eat. Although she may do all these things, and does not complain, she is grateful to have moments that she can share with her family. So in her world, a chronic illness is not a life sentence. It is an opportunity to think outside the box and live life to the fullest.

So who am I to complain if I have to work a little harder to lose weight or get pregnant, or if I have to change my diet? The bottom line is you have two choices: to surrender, or to fight. Those who know Makeda, knows she is a fighter.

I watch her fight to live daily, hence why I too won't complain. I simply will follow her lead and thank God for the opportunity to fight to live, by living an alternative lifestyle, which is a blessing, not a curse.

Journal Entries

I am sharing three of my journal entries as a 16 year old, so that you can picture what it may be like for a child experiencing a hospital stay.

Dear Mom and Dad,
 I am so scared. There was so much going and I am in so much pain. I don't understand why this is happening to me. This is so hard. I don't think these doctor's know what they're doing. No one is helping me. I'm trying to be brave but these doctors are mean and they don't want to listen to what I'm telling them. I'm going to doctor after doctor and everyone is saying something different. Nobody is really looking at the symptoms that I have. They are trying to tell me I have a disease from having too much sex, when I never had sex before. They just assumed that's the case. I don't un-

derstand how this can be. Now they are telling me I have to have surgery and I don't want any scars on my belly. I don't feel like I can trust them and I don't want to stay in this hospital by myself. Please don't leave me.

Dear Mom and Dad,
Today the doctors tried to put an IV in my neck without any pain medication. It hurt so bad I was shaking. They kept telling me to be still but I couldn't. They had me squeeze a bottle and hold someone's hand but that did not help either. After a while of sticking me three times with the needle I begged them to stop. I just couldn't take it anymore. They told me they were disappointed in me and thought that I should be able to handle it. Please call my doctor and let him know what's going on.

Dear Mom and Dad,
I really want to do well in school and make you proud. But this constant in and out of the hospital and getting cut all the time is really wearing me out. There was

so much going on all day and night. The lights, the bells and waking me up to see if I'm okay is driving me crazy. How many operations am I going to have I have tubes everywhere and they can't seem to figure out what's going on. This can't go on I don't want it to. I want to be a normal kid going to school with my friends, but instead I am stuck here in this hospital for months at a time. They have to keep changing the IV because my arms are so swollen. I don't know where they're going to stick me next. I hate this I have no more veins. Now they're telling me they need to give me a blood transfusion. I heard them talking and they said they felt sorry for me, no kid should have to go through this. I don't want anyone feeling sorry for me, I don't need their pity. I need them to help me get out of here. Last night I dreamt about food and eating. When I spoke to one of the nurses I convinced her to let me get some Dipsy Doodles from the vending machine. Don't be mad at her I didn't swallow them I just chewed them up and spit them out, wow that was the highlight of my day. Love You

Letter to My Parents

Dear Mom and Dad, I want to thank you for giving me life. I thank you for raising me in a family that was taught to love, be loyal and be encouraging regardless of the situation. You were persistent and consistent in trying to find ways to get me medical care and keep me alive. For the many days and nights that you worried and cried your eyes out because you were afraid that your child would die. I thank you for researching and giving me so many of the supplements to help my body heal itself. I am humbled by your tenacity to get second and third opinions and continue taking me to the numerous doctors' appointments and hospitalizations for surgery, even when they weren't covered by insurance. I can't imagine the trauma you must have felt thinking you would lose me every time. And as I read my journal and the one that Daddy kept I don't know if I could have handled this as a parent. I thank you for coming to the hospital at all hours of the day and the night trying to comfort me and call me with all of the different traumatic events that occurred. You were constantly advocating with all of the medical providers and administrators at the hospitals for room changes and Iv's that stopped working. You are my constant light and hope to make it, and for that I owe you everything I love and appreciate you forever

In conclusion, I have set some new goals to live my best life and continue moving forward.

Affirmations and quotes are a great way to speak positivity into your life. I find that you have to release anger, sadness and depression. It's only affecting you, your gut and your health. Don't waste time on the negativity or the negative people. They aren't worth your time. Released them and move on. How people feel about you is not your business. Sometimes this is easier said than done but you have to shower your body with positive thoughts and affirmations. The following are some of my favorites that I'd like to share with you. Many of them came from a book by Louise L. Hay called "Heal your Body." I read these several times a day.

It is with love that I totally released the past. I am free. I am love. I am safe. I trust fully in the process of life. Life is for me.

My thinking is peaceful, calm and centered.

I love and approve of myself. I am doing the best I can. I am wonderful. I am at peace.

I allow my thoughts to be free. The past is over. I am at peace

It is safe to let go. Only that which I no longer need leaves my body.

It is with love that I totally release to

past. I am free. I am love.

My intake, assimilation and elimination are in perfect order. I am at peace with my life.
I am safe. I trust fully in the process of life. Life is for me.

I express love and joy. I am at peace.

It is safe for me to live. Life will always provide for me. All is well.
(Hay, 1984)
A few quotes that pick me up that I assembled along the way.

I never lose, I either win or learn. Nelson
Mandela

"*Walk tall as the trees; Live strong as the mountains; be gentle as the spring wind and keep warmth of the Sun in your heart. For the Journey of where you once were and who you are now becoming is where the dance of life really takes place.*

Trust is like paper once it is crumbled it is very hard to straighten again. (Unknown)

*You are free to choose, but you are not free to alter the consequences of your decisions. (*EzraTaft Benson)

A dream becomes a goal when action is taken toward achieving it.

Bo Bennett

Accomplishments begin with the decision to try. Every job is a self-portrait of the person who did it.

Autograph your work with excellence.

Those who matter don't judge and those who judge don't Matter.

Elly Derr

What we resist, persist and what you allow to be; loses its power over us; for example fear and judgment of criticism.

Carl Jung

Cause and effect

Our energy radiates from inside out and has to pass through us before reaching others. We are therefore the first and foremost beneficiary of our own kindness and the first and foremost casualty of Our Own harshness such is the, Cause and Effect. I Love Therefore I Am (Abundant Lee)

The only way to do great work is to love what you do by Steve Jobs

We don't stop playing because we grow older, we grow old because we stop playing by George Bernard Shaw

Breathe in well-being, exhale your concerns *by Anonymous*

Summary

Life needs goals to look forward to in order to be meaningful. Life ain't over until it's over. I am establishing my new goals to keep me moving forward they are to:

1. Continue to be a successful servant leader. This includes publishing my book; reaching those individuals in need of service, and inspiring them to live life triumphantly.
2. Become a Global Leader
3. Inspire people with Chronic conditions to continue the fight.
4. Continue to model that life is not over with these tragic diagnoses.

And when these are accomplished, there will be more to come.

Acknowledgements

First of all I would like to thank Almighty God for continuing to bring me through these trials and tribulations. Secondly, I would like to thank my parents Harry A. Armorer and Dr. Audra Armorer for their love, care and diligence to protect me and get me the best care that they possibly could.

To my husband Jeffrey; Honey you have demonstrated unwavering support. Thank you for being a hopeless romantic. I know it wasn't always easy but you never let Crohn's be a burden. It's been one hell of a ride. Thank you for your love, support and encouragement. I could not have picked a better man and you obviously lived up to your wedding vows and all of your promises to give me a blessed and happy life with you.

To my three wonderful sons Jason, Jaron and Jafari; I thank you for keeping your eyes on the prize, for completing College and for doing all that was asked of you. I love you and I'm so proud of the men that you have grown into. You all make great role models. God bless you.

Thank you to my sisters Beverly, Gail, Ayshia and Sharifa who for my whole life took turns visiting, advocating, supporting and helping even when it was not easy to observe and you yourself didn't understand what was happening. To my brother Michael, finding you has given me a sense of completion. I love you and thank you for being a willing participant. Beverly you always did your best to keep my spirits up. I truly appreciate that because humor always helps.

Gail you visited, looked for natural supplements to help heal my body and cooked massive amounts of food for me and my family.

Ayshia you were my constant confidante and sounding board. You allowed me to voice the difficulties and have a pity party whenever I needed to.

Sharifa your support has been over the moon. Being the two youngest we were always together. You've held my hand through it all and continue to do so. If I was told that I wouldn't have to go through any of my trials and tribulations if I gave up my family; the answer would be an unequivocal no. I wouldn't change a thing I have the best family and I couldn't do it without you.

To my extended family you have truly been a blessing. Through all of my hospitalizations I can only remember one day when there wasn't someone coming to see me or support me. You are forever loved and appreciated.

To my special Sorors your love and support has warmed my heart. Simone Lowry you have fallen right in step and become family. I thank you for all that you have done and for being who you are in my life.

To my friends, I thank you for all of your support and encouragement. Thank you for putting up with all of my Crohn's humor and bathroom jokes.

To my sister Dorothy (Dot) Dorsey. I cannot thank you enough. You have cared for my family when I could not. You prepared meals, you dropped them off & you stayed with me at the hospital for days on end. There is nothing that I or anyone I know would not do for you.

A special thank you to my editing team who swooped in at the eleventh hour to ensure all was well. Thank you Aliya Stimpson; Gail Armorer and Ayshia Armorer. I could not do it without you.

As you wake up today, Remember you are created to succeed, designed to win, equipped to overcome, anointed to prosper and blessed to become a blessing.

Resources

Chiron-Institute
Dr. Sharifa Armorer, Practitioner, LCSW-R
914-384-3905
Web:www.Chiron-Institute.com
Facebook: Chiron-Institute

Dr. Melvin Grovit, Integrational Nutrition
15 Main Street
White Plains NY
914-633-1544

Dr.Robert Rosenzweig, Gastroenterologist
688 White Plains Road
Scarsdale, NY 10583
914-779-6200

Dr. Simon Lichtiger, Gastroenterologist
12 E. 86th Street, Suite 1

New York, NY 10028
212-831-4900
Dr. Harold P. Freeman, Surgeon and
Founder of The Harold P. Freeman Navigation Institute
55 Exchange Pl. # 405
New York, NY 10005
646-380-4060

Dr. Kevin Meacham
2071 Boston Post Road
Larchmont, NY 10538
914-834-4123

Pastor Hildred Reid, Prayer Warrior
Proceeding Word Ministries
P.O. Box 661091
Bronx, NY 10466
718-547-5451

Dr. Alexander Greenstein, Surgeon
5 E. 98th Street #1259
New York, NY 10029
212-241-8679

LINKS
CCFA: Crohn's and Colitis Foundation of

America
Crohnsandcolitis.com;
Chironsenses.scentsy.us;
Chrion-Institute.com;
NCTSN (National Child Traumatic Stress Network)

UOAA (United Ostomy Association of America)

Non-Invasive Alternative Treatment:
Acupuncture
Sound baths,
Angels and Butterflies Therapy for the Soul® Meridian Treatment (ChironInstitute.com)
Spirituality, Yoga, Vibrational Treatment
Floral Vibration Therapy (ChironInstitute.com

I would like to say in conclusion but this is a never ending story.
So ....
A Crohn's diagnosis or becoming an Ostomate does not mean that life is over. Neither of these situations is easy to accept initially. But as time goes on I im-

plore you to create a new "normal" and choose to live life triumphantly. My intention was to provide information, inspiration and an opportunity for you to see that you are not alone. This books purpose is to tear the shame off of having conversations about living with Crohn's Disease and/or an Ostomy.

Let us Coach you towards your Triumph.

Follow me on Facebook and let me know how you are doing. And remember to leave a review on Amazon.com
You can contact me at:
 914-837-4210
MakedaArmorerwade@gmail.com
On Twitter @*ArmorerWade*
On Facebook Crohn's Interrupted: Living Life Triumphantly
Website: Makedaarmorerwade.com
Blog: Crohn's Interrupted: Living Life Triumphantly
Instagram Crohn'sInterrupted_llt
#Crohn'sInterrupted
#Livinglifetriumphantly

Works Cited

Humor And Resiliency. (2013, Spring). *Crohn's Advocate Vol. 5 Issue 2*, p. 5.

Correspondence, C. o. (2016). Medical Events & Traumatic Stress in Children and Families. *Medical Events & Traumatic Stress in Children and Families* (pp. 1-47). Philadelphia: Children's Hospital of Philadelphia.

Crohn's Symptoms. (2016). Retrieved October 2016, from www.crohnsandcolitis.com: www.crohnsandcolitis.com/crohns

Hay, L. L. (1984). *Heal your Body.* Santa Monica: Hay House Inc.

Kuiper, N. A. (2012). Humor and Resiliency: Towards a Process Model of Coping and Growth. *Europe's Journal of Psychology*, 475-491.

Malabsorption Syndrome . (2016, October). Retrieved 2016, from Webmd.com: http://www.webmd.com/digestive-disorders/tc/malabsorption-syndrome-topic-overview

Nichols, L. (2016). Power Jam 2016. *Motivating the Masses.* Carlsbad .

Understanding Crohn's Disease . (2016). Retrieved October 2016, from www.crohnsandcolitis.com: https://www.crohnsandcolitis.com/crohns

Disclaimer: Any views expressed therein are mine alone and not necessarily those of the City of New York.

Made in the USA
Middletown, DE
02 July 2017